Survive Your Future With Chinese Medicine

RENE GORIS, PhD

Paperback: 978-1-969919-92-3
eBook: 978-1-969919-93-0
Library of Congress Control Number: 2025926829

Ordering Information:

Prime Seven Media
518 Landmann St.
Tomah City, WI 54660

Printed in the United States of America

Table of Contents

Forward: Purpose of the book....1

Introduction: How to use the book....5

PART 1....7

1: Why is Healthcare important?....9

How is that helpful?....32

Is it good enough?....37

2: The different approaches to medicine....45

The reductive method....48

Chemistry and authority....48

Industry and health economics....51

Health industry and pollution....55

Holism....70

Natural medicines and Holism....76

Tribal medicine systems....83

The best of all worlds....88

PART 2....93

Introduction....95

1: Future Risks assesment: What is the future we can expect?....97

2: Are we properly prepared? **107**
What do we know about the world, ourselves, and the future? *107*
Adressing my research purpose *108*
Risks of our modern medicine reality *113*
Lets review some relevant literature *117*
The research gap *126*

PART 3 .... **131**

The Daoland research project **133**
To test your health *133*
The computer game metaphor in health *151*

PART 4 .... **155**

Becoming a Daolander. How to make Yangsheng work for you **157**
Introduction: Global trends in natural health care *157*
Transformative health technology *169*
The Hierarchical Daoland diagram *181*
Rejuvenating health sports *186*
Rejuvenating Wellness/Care *199*
Daoland Culture Based Science Education *206*

PART 5 .... **211**

Daoland's art and science of becoming a professional human **213**
Introduction *213*
Daoland self-programming *223*
Introduction to causes *226*
East and west mutually influence each other *229*

Table of Contents

Forward: Purpose of the book *1*

Introduction: How to use the book *5*

PART 1 .... **7**

1: Why is Healthcare important? **9**

How is that helpful? *32*

Is it good enough? *37*

2: The different approaches to medicine **45**

The reductive method *48*

Chemistry and authority *48*

Industry and health economics *51*

Health industry and pollution *55*

Holism *70*

Natural medicines and Holism *76*

Tribal medicine systems *83*

The best of all worlds *88*

PART 2 .... **93**

Introduction *95*

1: Future Risks assesment: What is the future we can expect? **97**

2: Are we properly prepared? **107**

What do we know about the world, ourselves, and the future? *107*

Adressing my research purpose *108*

Risks of our modern medicine reality *113*

Lets review some relevant literature *117*

The research gap *126*

PART 3 .... **131**

The Daoland research project **133**

To test your health *133*

The computer game metaphor in health *151*

PART 4 .... **155**

Becoming a Daolander.
How to make Yangsheng work for you **157**

Introduction: Global trends in natural health care *157*

Transformative health technology *169*

The Hierarchical Daoland diagram *181*

Rejuvenating health sports *186*

Rejuvenating Wellness/Care *199*

Daoland Culture Based Science Education *206*

PART 5 .... **211**

Daoland's art and science of becoming a professional human **213**

Introduction *213*

Daoland self-programming *223*

Introduction to causes *226*

East and west mutually influence each other *229*

Modern Global Migration 230
Modernization 231
Exotism and revivalism 232
Yangsheng in a global perspective 239
There is only one study 243
To survive or to flourish 246
What we need and what we feel we need 248
Healthy and unhealthy conditions 249
Health study is the study of qi and dao 253
Life's habits 258
Good habits 260

PART 6 .... **275**

Daolands manual for the human geometry of life **277**
1 Size matters: maximize your form 277
2 The Dao of straightness 280
3 The Dao of roundness 284
4. Daoland principles of joint position 285
5 The root of breath 286
6 Apply in daily life and sports 288
7 Exercise and Aging 292

PART 7 .... **301**

My Seldon solution **303**
1: The research program 303
2: Focus on 3 skills 305
3: Becoming a professional Human 308
4: Learning time and epigenetic conditioning 310
5: Family management 313

6: Community building. *314*
7: The secrets of Composure *314*
8: Inner calm and health *318*
9: Solution building *321*
10. Solutions for city life *323*
11: Solutions for refugees *325*
12: Solutions for war victims *327*

FINAL **331**

Conclusions **333**
Conclusion and a words of thinks *333*

Forward: Purpose of the book

This book is originating in Wudang Daoist Yangsheng, which includes Daoist medicine, premodern and modern Chinese medicine as a whole, and all the things it contains from ritual, to exercise, massage, beauty and medical/mental healing. This book will show you also many leads to authors that have offered information that inspire this book. Much is originating with global concerns about peace, climate, and social harmony. The book is both a scientific queste, as well it wants to popularise a lifestyle of 'Social Activism', where you are the main tool for social progress. I call this the Hermit lifestyle. The Hermit is not always the person who lives in a grotto deep in the mountains. The hermit is a person dedicated to his or her purpose in life through a proces ogf 'meaning producing activities'. The term suggests that life in itself is 'Wilderness', and our life is a Grotto that we live in. It assumes that this life is the only life that is real to us now, and we try to make it work as good as possible following a wisdom of sorts. The wilderness is something we do not really control, but does affect us more or less, depending on how we live. And that we can control, so we should. How we live is how we biologically and socially generate health.

Unfortunately our world is nowadays very fractured. Overly focussing on keeping the books clean, taking an economic or business based approach to governance has gradually created a situation where the money havers want to set us back to a 19th century situation of Dickensian proportions. This world, which we can say to be ruled by ignorance at best and selfishness at worst, is getting out of hands, burdened by the consequences of how we actually live in contrast to what would probably be better for the most of us.

When I started living in China I saw the tail-end of Dickensian lifestyles in the world. What I learned is that it isn't fun if you are poor. But poverty isn't only a Chinese problem. It is a global problem and it is becoming bigger. Fortunately there is resistance against this situation. Unfortunately that resistance is badly organized and doesn't have enough power. And it will not untill it becomes a mass movement changing itself, so that wealth and power will feel ignored, and people do not need the dependencies on other peoples power anymore. This is what my Shifu You Xuande called the Taiji Lifestyle. This book helps you to understand it. A Taiji lifestyle is a pro-active lifestyle based on our natural needs, not our emotions and desires.

The main goal of any humanitarian person or humanitarian organization is to overcome the problems caused by abuse of economics and power, lack of education, and lack of health. This book is meant as a contribution to that agenda. Already as a child I was fascinated by the idea of human and animal rights. All living creatures individually are only living for themselves, but most creatures live in a relative timeless universe due to a limited consciousness. There is this sort of meshing kind of interaction between individual creatures and species, which we could determine as a form of swarm intelligence where species interlock to improve their own and their partner species lifestyles in their ecospheres. Individually animals and plants are aware of their needs, of birth, of aging, of gestation etc. But true is true, as human beings we can be so much more aware. But it all depend on 2 factors: Education and Health. Not on money or power.

This book brings these together and will offer you a handle to improve both, using the internet, community awareness, building ideals (Daoland is a realm where ideals become guidance), and building consistency.

This book introduces the depth of Chinese/Daoist 养生-Yangsheng (health care) in relationship to our will to control our health. We biologically have an imperative to learn to control our health by means of self regulating means to protect our health in aging and during and after a crisis of sorts. Yangsheng or life cultivation is nothing less than Natural Human Healthcare, or maybe in some ways DIY Healthcare (Do It Yourself Healthcare). Yangsheng is based on the idea of sub-health.

About 95% of people are sub-healthy, trending to good health or bad health. According to the World Health Organisation over 95% of the world's population has health problems. That is not a small amount. A 2013 study found that only about 4.3% of people worldwide had no health problems, so we can call these the super healthy. 62,4 are varying in health between 1 to 5 ailments. At the same time 33% of the population experienced more than five ailments. In the USA, about 6 in 10 adults have at least one chronic condition, with this percentage increasing significantly with age: over 90% of adults 65 and older, and about 75-80% of midlife adults (35–64) have at least one chronic condition. Across 24 OECD countries (Organisation for Economic Co-operation and Development), over one-third of adults reported living with a long-standing illness in 2021.

We all know what the long-term implications are from both trends. Upward is towards immortality and downward towards life degrading diseases and ending in death. So we can see that becomming immortal is smaller than 4,3%, while dying chances are more than 95%. Most likely you belong in the middle group. Yangsheng is focussed on this group to guide the trend upwards to stout health and immortality. DIY (do it yourself) is the guiding principle in that, the instructors and teacher are the support coaches in your program. The program has to lead to relative 'Health Autonomy'. The teacher want to coach you towards a neidan program. In a neidan program 'you are doing all the work'. You are then a self-alchemist, trending towards Radiucal Health Autonomy. The teacher also tries to support you to move away from ill health if you trend towards serious disease. When you are already aging, the teacher ties to guide you to restoration of youth.

This book tries to show you the need for self regulation in health in part 1 due to the increased list of threads of your health and life as well as of that of your community. Part 2 is introducting you to your health option in different risky situations, and it discusses the literature that inspires the reasearch, therefore it also introduces the questions we try to answer. In part 3 we go through some basic principles that keep us healthy and what happens when we deviate from this foundation.

Introduction: How to use the book

The book is divided in 3 parts. Each part discusses another angle. The first part does focus on our situation and the development of this book and the research it is part of. The second part is more practical. It gives you pointers that will work for you in all circumstances and it will introduce you to the content of the research project and how you will benefit from parttaking in it.

PART 1

1: Why is Healthcare important?

Discussing the need for Health knowledge to keep civilization civil

Over the long history of so called deep time, we have learned some things. In general both from sciences from different cultures, and the spiritual dimensions of these cultures, it has become clear that all civilizations are pretty much moral in nature, and based on cooperation. Nevertheless there are also bad agents. Situations can be so hopeless that conflict is the result. And there is also a small segment of immoral and amoral people that grasp opportune situations to improve their own lot without considerations for others. As a last category of bad agents there is the lack of knowledge and understanding that informs us well on limited data, but then the a-symetrical situation generates negative outcomes.

Another aspect we have also leaned that is that we as living beings do a lot of pattern recognition, which was previous considered to be intelligence. But pattern recognition is much like these puzzles with coloured dots that require a particular way of looking to see the underlying pattern. Originally these ideas were developed in art, through the methods of pointillism and impressionsism.

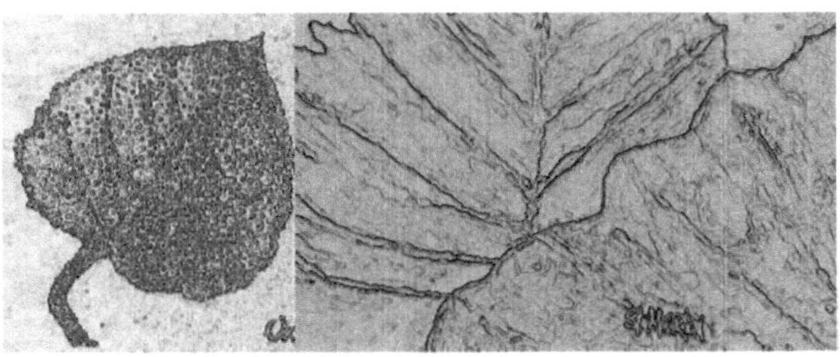

Pointillist and impressionist image of a leaf

Almost all our survival ability is based on pattern recognition. We estimate the chances we have to have a comfortable life. If we can make patterns reccur, we are able to feel more comfortable and thus generate habits. Habits take place in a safe space where we do not really pay attention anymore. In meditation and taijiquan we still focus on generating awareness space within habitual behavior to discover the depth of our actions. There is an esthetic value in that awareness. We also have learned that habits generate a sense of comfort. Habits are good tools to combat anxiety and fears. The secret of habits is time ordering. East Asian societies throughout history paid much attention to habit styles to generate order and harmony within society. The educationalist schools of Confucianism are especially focussed on ordering behaviour as a internalizing learning tool. It achieves that every person becomes a philosopher and acts directly from the heart with genuine commitment if they do right by the requirements. On a darker note, we find that even people continuously abused, get used to that habitual abuse, and learn to find forms of happiness. It is irregularity and unexpectedness that instills fear in our hearts. Regularity and orderliness gives a sense of safety. Chinese medicine and thus any form of healthcare based on Chinese medicine's ideas about reality therefore is about developing order in the way we live our life. Order helps us to establish health, where disorder upsets the biological and emotional system we call 'self' In addition to the orderlinessws we need for health and safety, we also need to have the freedom to do things that make you break out too, in case we need change to improve ourselves, or our world, as our world seems to be in dire need to do. The current order gives a sense of continuancy, safety to a degree, for many people, even the safety to create havoc to get our rude opinions through that reflect our self-dissatisfaction with how we got stuck ourselves in a deconstructive routine.

But if we are fair, we all know that that is not how we should do life. Life doesn't seem life threatening, even though for 87 million Europeans and many more globally that might change any second.

We all can understand that we should order our life in recognizable patterns, because it generates the esthetics of peace. If history let's us we will live our lives in peace. If not we will not, we should learn skills that comfort us. Habits of behaviour we can rely on and bring us peace and health.

When in frightening situations we require such a support, especially if we need to admit that the only person we can rely upon is ourselves, and that we can be the point person that is capable and willing to support others worse off then ourselves.

The material in this book, as rooted in Chinese medicine and taiji gongfu is to help you achieve this position of becoming the point person in crisis times, and to manage your own level of self accomplishment and health to find safety in any situation. The tool for this is the instilling of basic biological knowledge that can serve you as a healthcare. This book isn't going to provide you with all the tools you need, but it is offering some essential tools and insights. It is also an invitation to become stakeholder in my research as a participant, and from there perhaps even start a new career. The research is going to test a variety of factors from simple biofactors to behavioural factors and experiential factors to see how things will work out in an actual crisis. Something like this has nev er been done, and thus nothing is known about how natural medicine holds up in crisi, other than through anecdotical evidence. What the research tries to do is to develop reasons for governments and organizations, educational institutes from young to old, to change the way of providing healthcare and health education. In this book I am outlining much of the reasons for my research. I also do so on my Patreon channel[i] and on my Youtube channels[ii]

The question why healthcare is useful is a rather pragmatic one, because healthcare is 'useful', because it improves and maintains population health, enhances individual quality of life by reducing pain, increasing mobility, preventing premature death, and fosters economic growth through a healthy workforce and job creation in the health sector. It is also fundamental for social well-being, contributing to social cohesion, reducing health disparities, and upholding the human right to the highest attainable standard of health. In short: "Health is a civilizing agent".

When preparing for this book and my research I started posting on social media about it. Mohammed, a Rohingya refugee in Bangladesh contacted me, asking if I could adapt my program for his group of refugees. They are already for eight long years living in a forest with crude thatched huts. They did flee from violent prosecution from Myanmar, being a minority religion.

Many were killed, and Bangladesh did let them to stay in some 10 camps, 1.2 million refugees all together. There isn't much of healthcare or education for them, basic limited self governance only too. Rohingya refugee camps in Bangladesh are governed by the government of Bangladesh, which manages the response through administrative directives and works with humanitarian organizations like UNHCR and others. The system lacks a specific refugee law, so the government utilizes administrative instruments, while humanitarian agencies handle day-to-day services and have their own complaints mechanisms within the camps. Rohingya refugees have limited access to legal rights, education, and livelihood opportunities.particularly concerned about the safety of Rohingya refugees because of the materials used to make temporary shelters. Today still, there is worry because refugee families live in self-built bamboo and tarpaulin shelters. Many of these homes, built when the camps were founded, are now worn or degraded. The impact of heavy monsoon seasons, devastating fires and violence in the camps has repeatedly shown the need to rethink the approach to shelters and healthcare for refugees. Health is the most important thing, becasue health makes you more clear in your thinking, planning and doing processes.

This all illustrates the value of self preparation in many forms, but the ability to take care of your health and share methods among each other that do not make you dependent on external resources is clearly the most important. Health precedes the ability to create a civil social interaction, and cooperate calmly to organize and improve the general quality of life of a group.

In prehistory, success of any social group dependent on exactly these same skills. Common modern day 'end of the world preppers' are stashing to winter poor or destitute times, but it takes funds to prepare for that form of prepping. It is out of reach for most people. An underground bunker, food supplies, they might all be just out of reach during or after a crisis, and then you are left only with your luck, faith, and agression to get things done. More-over, they base their prepping on the nominal presence of the benefits of modern healthcare. These are gradually dwindling supplies.

Modern healthcare implies care by third parties such as therapists, doctors, surgeans, nurses, medications, digital support etc. Healers, holistic medicine people, natural medicine theraputics and cultural medicines to name a few, are commonly sidelined in regulation or severely restricted because they do not always fit the rules and regulations of modern industrial and evidence based science. They also often do not do more than supporting comfort in the run of the mill of modern organized city life. Unfortunately, due to past lawsuits the different approaches to healthcare are not considered equal. But they also didn't develop in a direction that necessitates their existence other than as an extra option in the same category as comfort food. A fair right to have but with limited usability, even though many people are helped to a great degree by their works. It is in no way that I say this as a complaint, but more to put things in perspective.

The common reason given for this situation is that modern science is "legally recognized" more than alternatives due to its reliance on 'a rigorous, evidence-based scientific method that emphasizes objectivity, systematic observation, experimentation, and replicable results, leading to consistent, predictable, and well-substantiated knowledge that underpins societal trust, technological advancement, and effective policy-making'. I have put this into brackets to emphasize the self validation that modern healthcare gives itself. Again, I do not want to criticize the good that they do, the problem is more in its cost effectiveness in relationship to that goodness, and also how it keeps people away from self management of health, even though that morally would be the best. Funding organisations often point out that outcomes from preventative healthcare can not be clearly enough measured. But that is not true ofcourse. It can be tested that preventative action can have solid outcomes or not on the shorter and the longer term. That is what the research I invite you to take part in is aiming to do. There is a short term plan, becasue that has to help me graduate. The graduation can help people like us to have a voice in policy making.

Daniel Keyes, et al reason in "Prevention Strategies[iii]" that the natural history of disease can be classified into 5 stages, namely 'underlying, susceptible, subclinical, clinical, and recovery/disability/death'. Corresponding preventive health measures are categorized into similar stages, allowing for targeted interventions at the relevant stages. For Chinese medicine in general the idea is that it is morally right to help yourself by being in a healthy starting point at any time of your life, to prevent diseases to occur as much as possible. Dependency on clinical intervention at any time can be costly. Healthyness includes being fully aware, having control over the motility of your body, and access to proper food sources. Keyes et al state that preventive measures include primary prevention, secondary prevention, and tertiary prevention. Gordon described these traditional stages of prevention as prevention, treatment, and rehabilitation, offering a clear and practical framework for structuring public health interventions. When clients come to me for help I allways first access which category they are. And you should do the same to yourself. It shows you the warning signs for what you ought to do, or better, that you ought to do something about yourself. In the Taiji yin-yang theory we say that a small force can influence a bit one, but best At an early stage of the appearance of the big force. A settled disease certainly habitually is a big force, difficult to influence. So curative therapies are sometimes needed but should be avoided where possible by taking care of your health before something happens to you. Preventative practice is a small force moving a bit one. My Daoist teacher Shifu You Xuande (master-father mysterious virtue), where I took my oath as a Daoist monk, explained me the principles of what he called 'Taiji thinking', which basically implied responsible action by knowing your future risks, like in the before mentioned 87 million Europeans constantly under thread of natural disaster and social conflicts.

Going back to Alternative medicine styles, their alternative viewpoints often lack this empirical grounding and systematic validation, making them less reliable and thus less acceptable within legal frameworks and society's understanding of truth and reality. Their on itself valuable insights are not taken in consideration within the safguarding of life and health. What is left out in this story are several factors. Often people fall back to concepts like "traditional", "intuitive", or "spiritual", without having a clear idea what these concepts mean. Traditional basically means commonly used, Intuitive means that you have derived this through long time experience within your box of understanding, and spiritual means that you think you have elevated ideas about things. That doesn't take away its value, but for science based researchers and practitioners that will not be sufficient proof. They might be willing to accept they are wrong too, but you need to proof it in their way.

Today, CAM practices may be grouped within five major domains: alternative medical systems, mind-body interventions, biologically-based treatments, manipulative and body-based methods and naturalism and culture based therapies. For instance, Chinese medicine is a medicine approach that dates back to 2500 years ago in written form. China, Korea, Japan, India and Vietnam have all developed their own unique versions of traditional medicine, strongly influenced by the Chinese medicinal sciences.

Alternative medicine is commonly categorized together with complementary medicine under the umbrella term "Complementary and Alternative Medicine", CAM in short. Complementary medicine refers to therapies that complement traditional western (or allopathic) medicine and is used together with conventional medicine, and alternative medicine is used in the place of conventional medicine. Alternative medicine refers to therapeutic approaches taken in place of traditional science based medicine and used to treat or ameliorate

disease. Chinese medicine and Ayurvedic medicine can be seen as alternative medicine and can be considered rather complete medicine systems by themselves. Both in theory and practice they do not need to rely on biomedical research. The relationship with biomedicine is forced upon them. Even though it nowadays drives innovation and understanding, it doesn't nesscasarily justify the involuntary nature of the arrangement. It would have been better if Chinese and Indian medicine systems could have volunteered to investigate biomedicine. They would have been allowed to understand biomedical results within the context of their own theoretical framings. They have their own scientific method developed over the ages, but not always as systematically deconstructed as the modern scientific method does. Xü Anlong in his 2022 book : "Yinyang You[iv]" points out that compared to biomedicine Chinese medicine, Chinese medicine in the past did not test its work in trials. Nevertheless it was experience based and well reasoned on the basis of its theoretical models. Thus it developed different approaches in medicine, such as alchemy as a foundation for first food medicine, and later in herbal medicine, but also for internal alchemy for deep understanding of food medicine, meditation, exercise etc. Natural or cultural medicines though, are focussing on experiental observation, and are as much empirical as biomedicine is. They are not anecdotical as many european herbal healers are by adopting the western biomedical analysis. They have let go of their root and are thus more a baloon in the wind than a natural health system. The main difference between natural medicine or cultural medicine systems, except judgements on what is what or how things work is that modern science uses an occult jargon that requires years of study to remember all the complicated nomenclature and what it refers to, while f.i. Chinese medicine uses a sense based language that is instantly recognizable as soon as you turn your attention inward. You do not need to memorize words, formula's etc, but you have to use your body and experience to memory map the theoretical system as a reality based program.

Acupuncture, massage, yoga, qigong, daoyin; they are the same as herbal medicine. You do need theory, but you have to embody the theory as well to comprehend the patterning and relations. There is also something a integrative medicine, which refers to combining complementary treatments with conventional care. But the root of it is always in the modern scientific method and thus a materialist perspective.

The basic philosophy of complementary and alternative medicine include holistic care, which focuses on treating a human being as a whole person. Self experience is usually a guiding light in making things holist. There are many hidden relationships between processes in the body. The discovery of the Jingluo (subcuteanal body flow system) is a good example for that. The Mainland Chinese writer of "Big Medicine (大药 Dayou)", proff Wu Guozhong[v], discusses the holistic principles of the body system by showing how body parts and organs can be altered by manipulation from unexpected angles. This principle is already known in East Asian medicine for milennia, and became summarized in the late Song dynasty as Taiji Therapy (太极疗法 taiji liaofa), (de)polarizing (taiji-ing) one part of the body, to affect another.

The actual research done in these medicine and health promoting approaches is done usually on the basis of western biological sciences and wants to be understood and adapted in this context. The amount of research done in this context is significant. But ideas about medicine from within its own science is neither validated nor often researched. In the culture of origin health is not always perceived in a similar way with our modern vision. Jingcheng Dong writes in 2013 in the article 'The Relationship between Traditional Chinese Medicine and Modern Medicine'.[vi] To paraphrase he made clear that in the present time there is a sort of symbiotic relationship in research between Chinese medicine and Western scientific methodology, acknowledging in his conclusion that this urges to the review of past knowledge for recognition which can fit into this modern science and which cannot. The emphasis is on proofing value on the basis of limited perceptions through testing and statistics. We also see that most research therefore is done on food and herb substances because they can easily be tested and described as chemical formulas. They get adapted based on the alternative determination of its compounds. The secret of Chemical formula is that they focus on one or a few controllable substances in an organic structure. There is an irony in this, namely that for instance a tree leaf contains hundreds or even thousands of distinct chemical compounds, including essential structural components like water, carbohydrates, and proteins, as well as vital pigments, minerals, and a vast array of specialized metabolites like terpenes, flavonoids, and alkaloids, which can vary significantly by species, soil conditions, and leaf health. Therefore testing for one or a few chemical substances doesn't really say anything about the actual biological structure and its effect on the body. This approach science takes is called reductionism. It cuts out the uncontrollable factors. Therefore logically it shows only partial evidence for the effects of a herb, but it allows for the production of artificial substances that imitte that effect, such as the vitamins in your vitamin shop. It is sad to see that many herbalists are now looking at the science determined foundation of a herb and allow for a machine logic of standardization.

Syed Amin Tabish wrote in 'Complementary and Alternative Healthcare: Is it Evidence-based?' (2008)[vii] that the use of alternative medicine appears to be increasing. A 1998 study showed that the use of alternative medicine in the USA had risen from 33.8% in 1990 to 42.1% in 1997. The most common CAM therapies used in the USA in 2002 were prayer (45.2%), herbalism (18.9%), breathing meditation (11.6%), meditation (7.6%), chiropractic medicine (7.5%), yoga (5.1%), body work (5.0%), diet-based therapy (3.5%), progressive relaxation (3.0%), mega-vitamin therapy (2.8%) and visualization (2.1%). In the United Kingdom, limited data seem to support the idea that CAM use in the United Kingdom is high and is increasing. Since that time these numbers have only increased and therefore more and more research is being done. Moreover, increasing numbers of medical colleges have started offering courses in alternative medicine. Accredited Naturopathic colleges and universities are increasing in number and popularity in the USA. They offer the most complete medical training in complimentary medicines that was available in 2008. In 2008 Britain, no conventional medical schools offer courses that teach the clinical practice of alternative medicine. The university based courses on offer all were Bachelors of Arts. However, alternative medicine is taught in several unconventional schools as part of their curriculum. Universities of natural medicine include the National University of Natural Medicine (NUNM), Bastyr University, Sonoran University of Health Sciences, and the Canadian College of Naturopathic Medicine. These institutions offer graduate-level programs in naturopathic medicine, which focus on holistic and preventative approaches to healthcare alongside the study of basic sciences. Some top universities for Chinese natural medicine include Beijing University of Chinese Medicine, Shanghai University of Traditional Chinese Medicine, and Nanjing University of Chinese Medicine. Other well-regarded institutions are the Guangzhou University of Chinese Medicine, Chengdu University of Traditional Chinese Medicine, and Tianjin University of Traditional Chinese

Medicine. These universities offer a range of programs focused on Traditional Chinese Medicine (TCM), and many have English-taught programs for international students. But all are rooted in Biomedical science education. Of all these mentioned universities and the ones I forgot, which one offers natural or cultural medicine it its pure form? Teaching is based mostly on theory and understanding of alternative medicine, with emphasis on being able to communicate with alternative medicine specialists. They do that by means of more and more obligation to adapt to the western medicine curriculum. Therefore they lose their scientific independence under that influence. PhD, Doctorate Investigators and Teachers like me have gone in resistance to that process, because it forces the eradication of much valuable to know. Much in this book for instance is about things which used to be common practice in Chinese medicine, but does not seem to have a place in modern medicine, partly due to that scientific adaptation.

Another aspect is that exotic languages are often based on western values. Amateur practitioners and writers often equate similarity with sameness. Andrew Chesterman for instance shows already in 1984 in a linguist study called 'Contrastive Functional Analysis'[viii] that "similarity isn't necessarily symmetrical", and he explains that "symilarity isn't necessary transitive either". The first means that word meanings do not need to mean the same. Take the word 氣 Qi, which is translated all too often as 'energy'. But energy translated in Chinese is '活力-Huoli'. This asymmetry means the translation is wrong. In the second case if energy would be similar to Huoli, and energy would be similar to qi, then it does not imply that qi is similar to houli. In Chinese Huoli is used for calory calculation in for instance fuel burning. Qi on the other hand is an indication of the quality of something. The similarity between things is suggestive of sameness, but in fact it can be misleading. In fact linguists suggests that similarity and sameness is a gradation of overlap.

Chesterman in 1984 suggested that similarity means two things share at least one feature, and sameness requires the overlap to be complete.

But let us make a bit of a bridge here. Because so far we talked of the differences between approaches to therapeutic work. Although it is interesting, that is not what this book is about. Here I wish to state that what is more important than either two of these: What you can do every day by yourself (the second part of this book is offering some solutions, as is the research program helping you to generate a full program to help you in this respect). In the remainder of this book we will make many sidesteps, but in the end we always come back to what you can do yourself. This book and the research associated with this book and its topic of "Surviving the Future" has to fool proof you against the errors of the industrial and therapeutic approaches of third party stakeholders.

With this book I point to you as a stakeholder in your own health, the health of your community, and the health of future generations. Whatever is introduced in this book is meant to give shape to true family health education that can be passed on from generation to generation, grow and develop over time and seed future civilizational development due to the humanitarian thoughts embedded in self regulation and self experience based natural healthcare.

Who is controlling your health

During the COVID crisis many people were caught off guard by the fact that the situation required by law that boards of medical decission makers were able to dictate policy. But in fact laws all over the world have been synchronized especially to let healthcare institutes take over applying all medical and legal instruments to control the epidemic outbreaks.

The World Health Organization was founded with the rights and obligations of governments and citizens in regard to health affairs. This Global approach has saved us many times without us even noticing. They often act pre-emptive. It was the COVID time just that the USA system and some other areas was rendered ineffective because of the abandonment of the support for the people by means of preventative supplies and capacities. This happened becasue of economic reasons. They wanted to safe on their budget. To be clear: to safe money in one branch of policy to spend it on something else that they prefered to spend it on.

The WHO website says:

> *"While disease outbreaks and other acute public health risks and events are often unpredictable and require a range of responses, the International Health Regulations (2005) (IHR) provide an overarching legal framework that defines States Parties' (countries') rights and obligations in managing public health risks, events and emergencies that have the potential to cross borders. The IHR are an instrument of international law that is legally-binding on 196 countries, including the 194 WHO Member States. They establish rights and obligations for countries, including the requirement to designate or establish Responsible Authorities; establish and maintain core capacities for surveillance and response, as well as at points of entry; notify to WHO public health risks and events with actual or potential international public health implications, regardless of their origin or source; verify information of*

> *public health risk and events of which WHO has become aware through informal and unofficial sources.*
>
> *The IHR set forth the obligation for WHO to maintain the global public health early warning function and to coordinate international response efforts.*
>
> *Additional provisions address the areas of international traffic, such as health documents for international travelers and conveyances on an international voyage. The IHR include important safeguards to protect individual rights in relation to the treatment of personal data, informed consent and non-discrimination in the application of health measures under the Regulations."*

In local provisions in governments there are also other limits to people's freedom installed, namely when your physical or mental health endangers you or your fellow beings. As such these laws are benign, but in some cases they can also be abused to take away freedoms unnescessarily, force lockdowns when other options are also available. The moral truth of decissions is sometimes hard to decipher. In every group of decissionmakers there will be elements that have only the best in mind, and some who have other motives.

In many countries, when somebody warns the authorities about your risky situation, that can be family, neighbours, and at least at some stage the police, the situation becomes a matter of law and a health care agent will be appointed to you, usually through the courts. You will have only limited rights of self determination. When you get medication, most medication are psychoactive, so they change your behaviour, just as your disease also changes you. Disease is a psychoactive agent. Fever can make you hallucinate. In fact many recreational drugs temporarily induce fever to make you hallucinate or feel better. Psychoactive medication, like your disease, works by temporarily altering your neurochemistry, which subsequently leads to changes in your mood, cognition, perception, and behavior. Both disease and medications interact with the brain through the body to produce these specific effects, causing the modification of the function of receptors, thereby affecting how a person thinks, feels, and acts. Well knowr psychoactive medicines are antidepressants: These medications aim to rebalance neurotransmitters like serotonin and norepinephrine, which are associated with mood regulation, helping to alleviate symptoms of depression. It doesnt become normal through. When using the medication longer time it feels normalized (ebbed), but medication never brings you back to normal. In fact it numbs you out for the disease caused pressures. Anti-Anxiety Medication work likewise. These often target GABA (gamma-aminobutyric acid) receptors to increase inhibitory signaling in the brain, reducing feelings of anxiety. It doesn't change your casues of anxiety, but it just makes the experience treshold higher, so that you can ignore it longer. But it all sounds rather abstract, doesn't it? It doesn't focus on the casue at all, but on the experienced effect. On the other hand, what is relevant to you is 'if you can be your old self', am I right? Chemistry is like an invasion force, and ditto it tends to hold your body hostage, while doing your body and your mind damage, and rather too often forces addiction onto you. The medication doesnt really cure you, but it represses the disease effect and replaces it with something else. The process of wheening off of your medication likewise can take some time, because too often the situation regresses to the original or a new health problem.

Most medications are in some form stimulants or depressants. A lot of their effect depends on the circumstances where they land. And it isn't just industrial medications that suffer this problem.

Natural medication does the same. In fact all you ingest does that. That is why a candy-bar or a beef-stake are easyer for you to get addicted to: they are more strong stimulants with more direct effect. They numb out other ingredients and their effects on you. These dominant food stuffs are hurried substances that immedeately change your mood. And their damage is their effect on your digestion.

Everybody nowadays knows that bacterias in your gut thrive on sugars, especially the ones that do damage because of quantifying exponentially and eating other bacterias in your gut. The story is that meat is very easy to digest. Carnivores have the shortest guts, for their mass, in comparison with omnivores, such as we humans. Our intestines hover between those of carnivores and herbivores, whom often have longer intestines and a longer predigestion tract. On average, transit through the small intestine, where digestion of meat mainly occurs & is completed, takes 14 hours. The small intestine breaks protein down into amino acids using trypsin, erepsin & other enzymes. It emuslifies fats using bile salts for uptake into the lacteal vessels. The small intestine is the only part of the gut that actively absorbs nutrients. The problem is that our digestion is not really very effective, so over time, especially in combination with sugar and spice intakes and medications, the meat gets stuck in the intestines, causing degradation of the peristaltic digestive system, and eventually causes constipation due to the fact that waste products get stuck in between the muscle and digestive tissues, sometimes causing (chronic) infections, and sometimes cellular damage and cancer. Foods that mostly cause infections are raw or undercooked meat, poultry, eggs, shellfish, and unpasteurized dairy products. Unwashed fruits and vegetables, contaminated water, and ready-to-eat items like deli meats and salads. Foods that often cause constipation include high-fat items like red meat and fried foods, low-fiber foods such as white bread and white rice, dairy products for some people, and unripe bananas. Additionally, excessive consumption of processed foods and sugary snacks, as well as high intake of alcohol (also a sugar), can contribute to constipation due to their low fiber and dehydrating effects. Doesn't sound good for the myths on meat eating by "meatarians" (people who think they are carnivores). Meatarians insist that meat eating is natural for people, especially raw meat. But why do you think you need to deworm your outdoor pet car on a regular basis? All meats contain parasites. Parasites kill us. So when we learned to make fire, and eventually learned to cook food, people experimented with the corpses they found and ate from when really hungry. They knew that meat eating is risky because of both the parasites and the risks for our digestion. They found that roasting the meat deeply reduced the risk for parasites, but not the risk for constipation. In Chinese cuisine meat is often cut in tiny pieces and is deeply fried with strong herbs to get rid of the 'dead animal taste' and reduce the risk of over eating on meat or becoming infestated by parasites.

In Chinese medicine we also say that in potential we can live for ever. But because of wrong lifestyle we become needy and greedy. The Daoist texts on diet in the "Cloud Coffer of Seven afflictions" (a compilation of texts from the beginning of the Ming dynasty / end of the Song dynasty on Daoist spiriotual and health sciences that I am translating) explains that we cannot live without compensation of that what we lose due to wrong lifestyles. We breathe and eat to compensate the loss, and the biology of our body cannot stop to ask for more. It says that eating and drinking can make us wise, but restricting food and drink volume can makle us live long. Only through breathing we can live forever. That isn't an easy process though. It takes a lifetime to correct our errors in lifestyle, such as emotional food preferences such as cookies, meat, dairy, spices etc. In this particular chapter it details the process we go through to get there when we stop eating and become breatharian. Only after about 70 days of strict fastiong we start noticing the first benefits, but even after 3 to 6 years we are building on the improvement process, that also leads to hefty physical changes, such as that the intestines become like tendons. The inner space and bacterial inner cultures have then vanished. It is another kind of biology. It is also through scanning the interior where you can see if a breatharian is cheating or not. I have done a 78 day fast once, and believe me, I started feeling good, but I looked more like a walking corpse.

Can you imagine how it is for 100 days, compared by someone suffering from constipation taking the urge to eat away because the body is filled with undigested food remains...And also how it affects your feelings and emotions. When eating less, constipation is much less likely to happen. The online Mayo Clinic will tell you that constipation is fairly common. A lack of dietary fiber, fluids and exercise can cause it, but medical conditions or certain medicines may be the cause as well.

You may or may not know it, but some people do not even know they are constipated, but they do notice swelling or pains. When the constipation blocks high in the intestine, there is enough space to let the dregs that do pass still sort of form. When lower in the intestines it might not, and then people think they have diarrhea. For the Mayo Clinic passing turds minimum 3x per week is not considered constipation. For Chinese medicine -if healthy- defecation comes by itself every morning before eating, this means there is no constipation and the intestines are clean. Also when there is not too much stuff coming out it means you probably eat not too much, and that is always the best, making having a healthy gut more likely.

This means that you also have some authority over your body and health, your mind, moods, and emotions. The way you eat isn't an exact science, but you can make or break yourself when eating and drinking. Everything you eat has some effect on your mind and/or body. You have to remember that for later in this book.

Law also influences you and your health in other ways. There are lawmakers in every constellation of countries that decide how food should be produced and processed before it gets into the shop. It is guaranteeing that the food you eat is securely dead. It is the reason why people started so much thought to machine thinking by calculating calories, proteins, sugars, vitamins and fats for health. Food industry as a capitalist endeavour has to comply with the law but they prefer to have control over every detail of what you eat. Both producing food and eating foods is highly politicized. Let me mention here the 'food souvereignty movements'.

The following is from "the Peasant journal" (2014). The article on Food souvereignty was written by 9 people, but i will summarize them by the first name, Marc Edelman[ix]. They wrote:

> *"Visions of food sovereignty have been extremely important in helping to polarize broad-based and diverse movements around the need for radical changes in agro-food systems. Yet while food sovereignty has thrived as a 'dynamic process', until recently there has been insufficient attention to many thorny questions, such as its origins, its connection to other food justice movements, its relation to rights discourses, the roles of markets and states and the challenges of implementation".*

Edelman is tracing the concept's origins to a Mexican government program in the early 1980s. In contrast, several of the other contributors echo versions of the established account that LVC 'first articulated' or 'mooted' food sovereignty in 1996 at the Rome World Food Summit. Still others take a sociology-of-knowledge approach to the origins question, linking the beginnings of food sovereignty to the globalization of the 1970s, the Uruguay Round of the General Agreementon Tariffs and Trade (1986–1994), the predecessor of the World Trade Organization(WTO) or the rapid concentration of giant seed corporations. Clear is that the food souvereignty movements are protest movements venting social engagement with how we nourish ourselves. This book is also rooted in such movement's idealism, taking a slight turn left from the Chinese medicine theory.

Chinese medicine, and especially Tao Hongjing (456–536 AD)[x] was of the opinion that food is medicine and that it depends on circumstances what you should eat. Herbal medications, tonics, etc, should only be taken in extreme circumstances. Herbs and medicines also are foods, but with a higher potency, and therefore they steal the thunder of our actual foods. That you may hope you never have to depend on medications is the general opinion of premodern Chinese medicine people.

A last factor is marketing. People try to sell you food and seduce you to buy their products. Marketing is a very powerful demon-like entity, that we are dependent on for information, but that uses psychological trics to make us feel particular things about the products. But in the old world we at least had some connection with our food. Due to hygiene rules all food or most of the food in many places gets wrapped up and we become isolated from the food when we want to buy it. To keep food "fresh" the plastic is saturated with a gas to serve as a conservative, and to make it look fresh and attractive. This way sellers continuously seduce people with looks, but not with touch or smell. In e-commerce that is even more so the case. We are completely separated from the products we buy. This is not dissimilar to the process of medicine distribution, which are secretive formulas for commercial reasons, and distributed through a doctor that shields the medicines with titles as to on the one hand serve as a distributor of life saving substances, and also as a guarantee for quality with it. Nonetheless, many clients are not satisfied with regular healthcare. Michel Foucault wrote in "Birth of the Clinic"[xi], -one of my favourite studies- how modern medicine grew into this situation of absolute authority over our bodies and health. There is a medicalized monopoly at work in this exemplified in food and medicine laws, that seem to give us freedom of choice, but also outlines where the boundaries are for us as individual to develop autonomy.

Martin J.Walker writes in "Dirty Medicine, the handbook"about the history of resistance against these forms of food and medicine authoritorianism, or as he calls it: "corporatism". Reading this book, you are reading into this resistance too. In my preperatory research or research synopsis, I have clarified that in the medical and political world the assumption is that after broad natural disaster or war things sort of will be as now, in that 'everything that was will be', and all the tools we now have, will still be available. But this book takes the darkest corner, a small but significant risk as its starting point. The worst can happen, or your country goes broke. You become a refugee, or you lose your house and have to go live on the street. You do not wish to become robbed, or drugged, or worse addicted. Or if you have a family with you, you want to have option to keep everybody well. You want to be the one that offers hope to the people around you. And this research and this book aim to support you in that with handy tools.

How is that helpful?

In the above chapter we investigated some angles of who controls your health, and we found that the medical industry, medicine producers, food corporations and marketing play a huge role in determining the course of your life's health.

In this chapter we go have a look into how these institutes are helpful in your succesful and healthy lifestyle.

I think most of us nowadays understand that overall health related to the food industry is a mixed picture. We see that there are some positive gains in areas like food safety and decreased consumption of items like sugar and salt. But then most of these are replaced by other sometimes dubious industrialized production based products. There are also some significant negative trends signalled, like increased consumption ofultra-processed foods and insufficient intake of fruits and vegetables by replacement substances such as smoothies and fat based products with fruity flavours. While some regions and populations are making progress in healthier eating habits, the widespread availability of unhealthy, convenient food continues to be a major barrier to improved public health. Foodlaws are unequal. Some countries allow GMO products, and others not.

Marketing keeps everyone thinking we eat healthy food. Nowadays, adolescents and children are considered as a substantial target market by the food industry. This makes marketers to target children and adolescents by designing customized food advertising and marketing campaigns. Even in the commercial healthfood market we see problematic trends.

With its focus on the quantity of production, often to the exclusion of other goals, today's commercialized food system is on an unsustainable course. The problem begins with and is driven by industrialized production of both crops and animals. Industrialization is a product of technological change, public policy, and, most recently, globalized trade. The lack of sustainability derives from reliance on the intensive use of nonrenewable and hard-to-renew resources—soil, antibiotics, fresh water, and fossil fuels, for example—but also from the waste and pollution created by the industrial model. But people need food, so there is a guarantee for buyers, nonetheless there is a need for profits, so production expenses are lowered, substances are replaced by cheper substances and marginally over the last 50 years the rpoduction did creep to lower and lower production quality. Measurably a natural crop of salad might hold the same components as a natural one does, but still, its function as a container for nourishment value has decreased. If a snail has the choice between a natural plant or a crop of industrial salad, it will take the industrial salad because it is easyer to digest than a natural salad. That is also why farmers spray industrial products to keep what they call pests away from their crops. These added poisons end up in you, but also in a lot of other animals and plants, because chemicals are not selective.

In a 2009 article for the 'Journal of Hunger and Environmental Nutrition', David Wallinga writes that there are two sides to this situation: One side is the epidemic of obesity-diabetes (among other rising chronic diseases) and the huge future costs they portend. Medical costs of obesity in the United States are estimated as $147 billion annually, and climbing. Combined with other diet- related chronic disease (cancer, cardiovascular disease, stroke, and diabetes), that figure could be as much as 5 times higher. Another side is that there are more and more outbreaks of foodborne illness, food contamination scares, volatile food prices, and "food deserts," not to mention drought and water shortages, soil depletion, climate change, fishery collapse and other events with significant, but not always direct impacts on nutrition and health in our lives. Clearly, both food and health systems are under stress, and as a result our life is too. These are significant signs also that the climate isn't well, becasue the climate also relates to the quality of land. Shortage of water, desertification, growing asphalted surface volume, urbanization etc, all contribute to locally small but globally remarkable influences that we can nowadays see frequently in the news.

I do not know if you every heard of the ANTi (Access To Nutrition index)? Their index is assessing how the world's largest global food and beverage (F&B) manufacturers are contributing to addressing malnutrition in all its forms. They show that roughly 34% of the combined sales of the top 30 companies, are derived from `healthier' products. These top 30 companies are representing 23% of the global F&B market. A lot depends also on where you live. The least healthy products are being sold in low- and middle-income countries. They mark a slight silver lining. They say that this represents a marginal increase from 27% in 2021. If we could assume this pace of growth moving forward we would arrive at around 50% of sales derived from healthier foods at some point in early 2032. That implies ofcourse that we are greatly under served with proper nourishments within their own framework of thought and corporate science. Martin Ja Walker points out that corporations play the long game, in that they design pathways for products a long time before they come into the market. When the Dirty Medicine Handbook came out in 2011 we saw the first signs of a growing supplement market, which now is so big that people who are being told to have shortages of substance A or B they supplement this with another industrial product, that is all but medicalized. Some countries have supplements already medicalized.

We see the problem coming: a gradual degradation of food quality over time, compensated with artifical compensators. Let's name a few examples. Like bitter lemon and tonic water. Bitter lemon got its bitterness from Quinine. Quinine is a medication used to treat malaria and babesiosis. But untill beginning of this century it was a common ingredient in tonic and bitter lemon to give it its bitter taste. The good thing was that it therefore also was a fever repressant, or at least it resolved many infectuous fevers. In Chinese hospitals they used to let people drink a few liters of tonic water before they make x-rays of the bladder, or if they wanted to look inside, becasue it presedated the bladder and the body. Nowadays almost everywhere the quinine is removed and replaced with an artificial taste to control the quinine market/ Yellow sulfer used to be a general anti-infection medicine. You shouldn't take too much of it, but small quantities are quite good for you. It used to give colour to custard puddings. I used to proscribe it, to make it without sugars, because it was a wonderdrug against intestinal infections. Unfortunately it was removed from the pudding and replaced by corn powder and colorite. It made custard pudding a nuisance, and only attractive for kids for its sugary content. There are many products like this.

The University of Maryland, USA, has a database of natural ingredients. It mentions that Peppermint (Mentha x piperita) is a popular flavoring for gum, toothpaste, and tea, also serves as a calming agent to soothe an an upset stomach or to aid in digestion. Kids get it to soothe car sickness, because it has a calming and numbing effect. Thus it has also been used to treat headaches, skin irritations, anxiety associated with depression, Irratable Bowel Syndrome, nausea, diarrhea, menstrual cramps, and flatulence. It is also widely used to treat symptoms of the common cold. Mint's main component is menthol. Mint candies sometimes contain derivatives from plants such as peppermint oil or spearmint oil, or wintergreen from the plant genus Gaultheria. However, many of the most popular mint brands citing these natural sources nowadays contain none in their ingredient list or contain only trace amounts. All in all it becomes less and less possible to use these industrial products based on healing properties of plants or minerals, and from which they derive their name, for self-treatment. Corporate entities are blocking of the roads towards health through affordable inroads and solutions. They do not like us to tinker with their products, if that means they lose sales in more expensive medications, such as Quinine in Malaria medication or Sulfur based products for Irritable Bowel Syndrome.

Therefore, the question if food and medicine industry are helpful for our health, and or food security is one we cannot answer positively. And true too, living in large urbanized areas where people also control that plants in parks are mainly decorative and non consumable, or by washing away information about the edibility or healthiness of tree leaves such as from Oak, grapes, apple tree, hazelnut and so on.

What we learn from all the above is that for personal and communal security we need is a dual system of healthcare: the modern sciences and alternatives for life as it goes, but also something more simple and perhaps even tribal that we learn at an early age and maintain throughout life, and that we eventually can share with our children. Not so much just survivalism such as how to build a shelter, how to make fire, how to protect ourselves, or how to cut a tree. These things are of unbelievable importance to know. What we need is a self-management of health, focussing on preventing disease and maintaining health, that can be used as a foundation for other therapies as well. I am sure that knowing how to secure our health will organize society differently, and will less opportunity for social and crosscultural conflicts to rise, as well as that we become less easily victim to the sales people providing us with seductive but unhealthy products.

Is it good enough?

The research project started before I completed this book. After many years and testing things I found in my first PhD research I concluded a few things. But let me start from a beginning, because I did my research based on my interests in Daoist culture and medicines. For this I did a minor at University of Amsterdam on the History of Western Esoterics with Proffessor Wouter Hanegraaff and his team, since that the recent history is playing such a large part of modern Alternative Medicine methods, and has also infitrated much of modern medical mythologies in how doctors explain their work to their clients (like suggesting something is in your brain, imagination, or genetic). It also allowed me to rethink what I learned about Chinese medicine. I did resource research at Boston and Birchwood University libraries in the USA, involved myself with Chinese medicine organisations in Europe, and leaders in the field in the USA and Europe, and I moved to China researching for 13 years, following Daoist masters, Chinese medicine professors in Hubei, Sichuan, Beijing and Shanghai, studying their skills from microsystems to using large needle formulas (300 needles or more), single needles methods, a dozen of massage approaches in China, herbal studies, herb collection studies, etcetera. I got a lot of help studying Daoist and medicine classics, Yijing etc. I also got sideways involved with people from the national Chinese medicine government and their meetings on the future of Chinese medicine, and where I was also allowed to share my ideas sometimes. This I owe to the opportunity Dr Yang and Mrs Kong from the

Chaoyang medicine clinic offered me to test the educational model with Chinese medicine practitioners. Meanwhile I had my clinic and school in Amsterdam, that i often used as a testing ground and experimental laboratiory. Therefore, at periods I had to go back to the Netherlands to earn the funds to finance my research by myself. I had nobody supporting my research at the time. My students and participants support my research by paying for classes and therapeutic treatment. Some gave me donations. I graduated at IOU Foundation, nowadays part of Aztec University in Mexico City. The current director of the foundation, proffessor Sandra Hurlong, herself an antropologist, is still a good friend. My motivation was largely driven by the success I had by using these methods for myself. As a child I was born with a serious Kidney disease that would likely have got me on an artificial kidney before my 10th. I was fortunately enough to get an operation of 4 hours when I was 9 years old, just before my kidneys would fail. The professing Surgeon dr Wierdak, already diseased unfortunately, scraped one kidney clean from infections, and hoped the other would heal itself. That didn't really happen. From scans over time I found out that one got totally shrivelled and the other one only partly works. For this reason alone there was the need to manage my health very carefully and minimize impact while maximizing output. From this all I found Daoist health practice is the most economic one, and that motivated my research.

Daoist health practices are effective and allow for much leeway to minimize need for resources, control impact etc. It kept me away from needing medical support for the most part of my life. If I come it is to ask some questions. I didn't need any medication or treatment since I was 15, now 47 years ago. So I guess what I learned works. Anyway, in the operation I got into a coma due to oversedation: I kept waking up during the operation, opening my eyes and trying to sit up. I don't know, that is what they told me. They told me to never do any sports, but I liked exercise. I was doing gymnastics, but they strictly forbade anything that could pressurize my kidneys. He also told me when he retired (I was fifteen and got regular checks up to that moment) that it was unlikely I would live past 40/45 years old, which at the time I could not comprehend. When I asked him If I could do yoga or qigong when I was 11, he didn't know what they were, and as far as he knew he considered them low impact activities (which they can be). This sounded to me as a permission, which I widened also to taiji and taijigongfu, yingong, daoyin, application practice, experiments with food and medications (including sometimes poisoning myself by accident), all interrupted by 5 years of excessive drinking drug use and smoking when I was in my late puberty and early twenties. When I noticed my kidney issues returning (while also my liver was aching) I fortunately found the strenght to change my ways and get back on track. When writing this I am about 20 years past my presumed expiration date. In that period i also accumulated much knowledge from people teaching me, science articles, books, research etc, gradually getting met to this point.

To be quite frank: I usually advocate against summarizing or simplifying skils and understandings. I think we learn through saturation, not by means of simplified examples. Too many people offer simplifications rooted in the gist of what they think they learned. For some that will work, I am sure of that, but it doesn't provide the kind of people able to transmit a quality to the next generation. So to work as I do, you will need at least 5 years of practice for 10-12 hours a day. That is a lot to ask even for olympic atletes I understand. For this book and the research participation there is no such need. To become a proficient healthcare worker in the Daoland program some 2-4 hours aday of practice will get you far. You do not need to be great at things, but you need to understand a lot. But when in crisis, you only need a few skills, that is what this bpook and the research are about. If you do feel inspired to get ambitious, and you do want to become a master, do not get fooled, you do need a lot of time, do not let yourself be fooled that you can develop mastery of anything for only 10 minutes a day. Making that step isn't something you also can choose. Participating in a basic program as in this book and the research you make a choice for.

Either because you need to improve your health, or you see the need to have these skills in case you need them, or you just like to learn these things as a novelty, any reason is why you can decide to do it and complete it. But to do the whole thing and become a master (a Master Master, not a Bachelor-Master master, then the 4 hours/day will suffice) you best give up on having a social life, doing things for fun etc. And after that you will still have to keep dedicating yourself to practice and study every day. Skills are an aquired quality, but also need maintenance. Everyday your body learns new things, and that what you do most is what it specializes on maintaining. If that is learning Taijigongfu, or eating cookies, or drinking beer, or study farming, your body will help you whatever you do most to be maintained. So if you do bad things for your body, the body will help you make it worse. In Chinese medicine that is a function of the "Po", envoys accompanying you originating from the earth.Daoism says that they rapport to the god of Earth every month if you behave well, and the god of earth reports it to the god of Water, who determines your faith (that is why Chinese springfestival is so important to the chinese: it is when the new karma goes into effect). Do bad things and the Po and the Water God will make your body age faster, get sick or get damaged. That is ofcourse for most people just a bedtime story. But please remind yourself also that Biology doesn't have hollidays, weekend, parties or anything like that.

And you should also prevent that you become a fanatic. That kind of stress blinds the heart and the mind. Every thing you do is teaching something to your body: lazyness, pressure on your joints, polluting your blood, having negative thoughts. Chinese medicine points to your self-responsible behavior, as a species we have this to nature, the planet: respnsibility, because everything we do has an effect, cumulative.

So is it enough what I did for my health? A daoist wisdom says about food: "Eating can help you gather wisdom, eating a little every day offers you a long life, being able to survive on no food makes you an immortal." So I see myself aging in spite of my study. You judge when you meet me as part of the research participation how I do.

But what I have seen over time is basic principles of care for health. There are 13 different skills that people need to master:

1. *agility through fast qigong:* Wudang gongfu fitness is a fast mobilizing and strenghtening practice that done in moderation can help anyone to become liberated from tensions and locked joints
2. *balance as source of strenght in moving daoyin:* This slow walking practice knows different grades of complexity and bodily interpretation to achieve a deep sense of balance when moving in complex ways and how to develop strenght from there
3. *internalized allignement and finetuning in standing daoyin:* Many postures cand be used for this internal allignement practice to help you shape the interaction between bone form and muscle form.
4. *initial breathwork:* to produce internal circulation to regulate yin-condensate and yang-steaming as a means to generate focus

5. *advanced breathwork:* this skillset allows you to inwardly become fully self reliant, and to control senses as layers to conciousness
6. *external symmetry through qigong:* Qigong uses symmetry to reallign muscles and channels, and free up blood vessels, harmonize tensions and build inner peace.
7. *internal symmetry through regulation form and location of organs:* meditative exploration of the interior as a root for further peace and preparation for chinese medicine practice and understanding of the wuxing (5 consumers) theory framework.
8. *external a-symmetry through taijiquan meditation and applications:* Taijiquan brings a lot together lerned in the other skills, and teaches to weave these skills through the assymetry of life that is continuously polarizing our biology and mind
9. *self-massage:* This qigong stimulates your outer surface as if a masseur does that, emphasizing the inner order through its activities, separating in 3 different 50 minute sequences.
10. *food medicines*: through selective food testing understanding the underlying qualities of food stuffs and how they affect you. It is also foundational to learn for every herbalist that wants to understand Chinese Ingestive Medicine Theory. It also allows you to understand the medical quality of anything you eat.
11. *basic body geometry orienting meditations:* Directional breathwork techniques that have to connect your inner experience with the outer environmental mandala.
12. *anti-aging principles in self-care:* diverse meditations and simple massage and needle techniques to offer fellow beings general revitalization options, such as for digestive and yang issues of the body, casuing overweight, aging, and indirectly diseases.

13. *basic natural theoretical framework as a worldview*: This is probably the most important part, because there is nothing that works if you do not have a theoretical framework or worldview that binds all aspects of life together and gives you a sense of direction, destiny if you will about what you want to aspire to achieve. Idealism if you want to call it like that.

These skills are based on what I found in Daoist medicine theories and practices from pre-modern sources and traditions that have largely been taken out that what people call TCM (traditional Chinese Medicine). You see that people sometimes recombine aspects of this in programs, but often the theories of each of these activities are not forming a holist unity. The Daoland program I developed with help of all my supporters, such as teachers and students, is all based in a single theoretical graded framework. Doing the one and getting good at it, gradually makes you ready to also absorb the other skills in the same theoretical framwork, bound togeteher by the same theoretical goal. They do not garantee you immortality, but they should get you quite far on the way. Ofcourse there are always erratic circumstances, so please do not shoot the messenger, me, just try to understand the options it gives you. It basically shows that all actions in your life can be geared to certain results. In so far as we need to gamble on outcomes, it makes the gamble less risky if health and long happy living is your goal in life. If that is not your goal but you give this program a chance, you might change your mind, and gain much optimism about the world and yourself, inspite of the dangers around us. But then an optimism with eye for reality, and not the Austrich behavior (putting your head in the sand) we too often see ruin nature, climate, and society.

To make clear, this above listing is by no means everything. It just is the miniumum to maximize your chances to have a long and healthy life. But there is a bare minimum too. And this bare minimum can be learned quite easily by everyone to improve health, to maintain health, support food security under all circumstances, and train your alertness and awareness of your environment and yourself. That is what this book is intending to help you start with implementing, and to extend that practice by learning the skills in the Survival Healthcare program my research investigates.

In the above list these are nr 1, nr 10, and nr 11. These are Taiji gongfu fitness, Food medicine practice, and Dantian meditation in the Daoland program I over time developed. These skills can all be learned in about 3 months time given each of them some time every day. I'd say between 1 hour to three hours depending on your ability and dedication. In the research I monitor people through the learning process, the retention process and the implementation stages, to proof its viability. As skills you need to make them part of your being and behavior to be able to improvise when you need them. The second part of the book deals much with the underlying principles of posture and movement in this Daoist Health Care oriented program. And no, you do not need to become a Daoist to have use for this program. This program is to compensate for the lacks of civil health education in modern societies. Although I will have to explain some specific Daoist ideas not present in our western languages and scientific acceptance. They just add to your meaning. I hope they will help adjust how you see yourself and how you can improve yourself.

2: The different approaches to medicine

Medicine as a professional field cannot be called a standardized field. There are many different approaches available, and there are even different scientific methods. East Asian culture had its own scientific method. The Joseph Needham Institute[xii] has already for many decades been publishing books in which they discuss the variety of sciences and methodologies from China. Due to the colonial period much of this has been dismissed as non-scientific.

In spite of this judgement the Chinese people had discovered the magnetic compass, and used it to find an an auspicious location for graves as well as mapping their environment. They did discover gunpowder, and made primitive missiles as fireworks with it. Near two thousands years ago a scientist invented a seismograph, able to predict earthquakes. They developed mass production of earthenware, irrigation installations, the printingpress, the water clock and many other marvels for that time. Many inventions were seen as dangerous for social cohesion and therefore never mass promoted. Chinese culture was pretty conservative as a mercantile state. A mercantile state is a state that serves as a company with the king or president at its head. In mercantile states you can only do things with authorized permissions from highest up. Let me give you though one more example of scientific accomplishment.

In the Mozi, written by Modi (475-221 BC) we find several statements concerning force and motion. There is the statement, "Force is what moves a body." This may sound simple at first but is a statement at the foundation of modern science. If you slide an object on a smooth surface, why does it continue to move after it has left your hand? Your hand is no longer in contact with the object and no longer exerts any force, yet the object continues to move.

Another well known example: Suppose you pull a box across the floor with a string. There are several different forces acting on the box in various directions. A physicist examines the net force acting on that object. The scientist will sum-up all the forces in a particular direction to arrive at the net force in that direction. Now in the case of our box, the string pulls in a direction opposite of that of the friction produced by the floor. When two forces act in opposite directions and have equal magnitudes, the result is a net force of zero. If the horizontal component of the tension in the string is equal in magnitude to the frictional force exerted by the floor, then the net force acting on the object in the horizontal direction is zero. How can the object move if the net force is zero and we believe the statement that force is what moves the body? This is also a problem we face in our body due to the complexity of out muscles, bones, tendons, flesh, and fluids, that all cause friction when not practiced frequently or the right way. But anyone who has studied some physics understands that the object be it a box or a muscle or bone continues to move after it is released because of inertia, and this is in keeping with Newton's laws of motion. In the case of the object pulled by a string, we again encounter Newton's laws and the idea of acceleration. Since the net force acting on the object is zero, it has no acceleration and continues to move with a constant velocity. All this discussion of motion, acceleration, and velocity requires us to mathematically define what these quantities mean. We observe a moving object in class and then create mathematical terms that can be used to describe its motion. In fact, the Greek philosopher Aristotle struggled with the same questions and came up with answers that were inconsistent with Newton's laws of motion. Perhaps what this shows is a more universal idea of how the observation of natural phenomena spurs thinking people to seek more detailed explanations that ultimately give rise to scientific thought.

From here, we move into the subject of kinematics. Studies in kinematics are about the discussion of the energy associated with moving objects and the principle of the conservation of energy. This topic is typically introduced to students in physics by analyzing the motion of a ball thrown straight up into the air. The analysis becomes far more interesting when the object is a 200 kilogram fishtail percussion drill bit used to drill for salt brine in ancient Zigong. The area of Zigong has a long history in ancient China. Few people in the Western world know of the ingenious system used to drill salt and natural gas wells some 2,000 years ago. The ancient Chinese drilled wells that produced both salt brine and natural gas. Natural gas was used to fuel burners placed under pans of salt brine. Once the water was evaporated away, large salt cakes were formed. Salt provided a very lucrative commodity and became a vital part of the Chinese economy.

Chinese science is most emperical in its approach and very much focussed on finding practical applications. It doesn't spend much time on theorizing endless calculation methods as we do in the west. Evolution of technology therefore is gradual, but it also isn't theoretical. But do not forget: western science is also based on an empericism of sorts. In philosophy, empiricism is an epistemological view which holds that true knowledge or justification comes only or primarily from sensory experience and empirical evidence. Episteme is the knowing of phenomena. Empirical proof is what is verified by sensory observation and is repeatable. So, seeing an alien is not emperical proof, an alien appearing in a crowd and giving a lecture is empirical proof.

Let us briefly discuss some science related approaches.

The reductive method

The term "reductive method" in science can have two meanings:

1) A chemical reaction involving the gain of electrons or a philosophical. In chemistry, reduction is when a molecule or atom gains electrons, lowering its oxidation state, and is always paired with oxidation (the loss of electrons) in a redox reaction.
2) A methodological approach to breaking down complex systems. In the philosophical and methodological sense, scientific reductionism is the approach of understanding complex systems by breaking them down into their simpler, constituent parts.

When we discuss our health, or how best to survive in a crisis situation, we usually use the 2nd method. From this we understand that all people are by nature scientists. We study and discuss the sciences of life in informal formats. When facing a difficult situation we have to learn categorize what we go through in sort of a priority lists. This in itself is already a reductive method. The least important things on the list might in some situations even be discarded. It is hard to get more reductive.

The Chinese thinker Zhuangzi, living in the late 4th century bc, discussed bamboo. He asked how small you should cut Bamboo where it becomes less than bamboo: showing his awareness that things are often composites, and that if you reduced them enough they become something else.

Chemistry and authority

In modern medicine the authority of treatment is largely put on the chemistry of a problem. Emerging in the early decades of the 19th century, modern chemistry, organic synthesis in particular, played a major role in the evolution of science by providing molecules, natural or designed, for further investigations and applications. Various enterprises, most notably the dye and pharmaceutical industries, relied heavily for their establishment and advancement on discoveries and inventions in organic synthesis. During the nineteenth and early twentieth centuries, this discipline remained for the most part an isolated science in academia, whose practitioners were interested primarily in advancing it for its own sake through discovery and development of new synthetic reactions and their applications to natural products chemistry. The latter were considered as targets for structural elucidation and total synthesis. This paradigm changed significantly in the second half of the twentieth century when a number of investigators turned their attention to producing sufficient quantities of scarce natural products for biological studies and medical applications. In Chinese medicine we see something similar happening. During the Song dynasty (960 to 1279AD) Medicine, and especially herbal medicine was taken away from the Daoist practitioners and received status as a literati art/science. Developing recipies became a skill. For a thousand years it was common to keep formulas simple. A recepy with 1-5 herbs was very common. Hua Tou's "Shennongbencaojing" (the agricultural god's classic of herbs) classifies herbs as having Wuxing values. These are five taste related qualities, but they were also classified for 3 categories of people: The very ill, the nominally healthy/ ill, the extremely healthy. You may remember the population distribution of health we discussed above. The Song literati were assigned with the task to show their superiority over the foregoing Tang dynasty doctors, so they added 10 or more medicines to the recipies, where the medicine had to often neutralize each other due to the dangers caused by complex formulas. This method is also used by modern Chinese medicine, for whatever kind of reason, but the effectiveness of herbs is based on the authority of modern western chemistry.

Following the discovery and development of penicillin as an antibiotic, the pharmaceutical industry intensified its activities in the isolation and development of natural products as drugs while at the same time it began to exploit the increasing power of organic synthesis to design, synthesize, and test small organic molecules as potential drug candidates through what became known as medicinal chemistry. The process of rational drug design based on the identification and validation of a biological target followed by medicinal chemistry to find small molecules that would bind and modulate the function of the biological target became the standard paradigm for the drug discovery and development process during the last decades of the twentieth century. At the same time, chemists and biologists in academia began to recognize and appreciate the importance and potential impact of merging their efforts toward the elucidation of biological pathways and disease pathogenesis. It is this pathway that nowadays guides modern TCM, while in the past medicine was ruled by empirical proofing, and for this the medications have to stay simple. In the research we use a method based on the Shennongbencaojing to help you find out the qualities of the herbs and how they influence you. There are as mentioned 3 grades:

- medicines that can be ingested riskfree and belong to heaven and is the king herb
- medicines that might be toxic and belong to nature and is the minister herb
- medicines that are toxic and belong to earth and is the envoy herb

A formula has usually one of each to harmonize the person to the whole of reaality. What medicine you need depends much on your individual situation. The secret of herbal medicine is that you have to look at food as medicine, and herbs as special medicines that add to your food. It isn't difficult, you only need practice to take authority over your health back. That is practical for many reasons. Especially in times of crisis. Designing a dish for lunch, breakfast or dinner can be done along these lines.

Industry and health economics

The economics of the health industry are the motivation for the providers of healthcare, and it stands in a triangle with insurers and patients, where the patients are both costumer and product, providing billions of revenu, holding costumers in many countries into what I interpret to be a financial stranglehold. The industry and insurers are both stakeholders in mainting a status quo, as well as developing a growth market. That approach also makes it vulnerable, as an industry, especially when disasters strike, and they have to rely on government funding to maintain service as good as it goes. Industry survives by maintaining a statusquo. Every now and then a new method is being invented and that method might be disruptive. But however disruptive that method is, it can be managed in the same economic framework. For us as consumers of medication it means that we are kept on economic leash, which consumes part of our income, especially when our health is failing, such as when we are aging. In a way, and industrials will not be happy when anyone says this: economy is a parasitic entity. It isn't scientific.

Ted Gioia is a music critic and historian whose musings tend to wander all over the cultural landscape. In an article titled "Are

We Now Living in a Parasite Culture?" Gioia explains here that "Nowadays, parasite businesses are the largest corporations in the world. Their technologies do many harmful things, but lately they have focused on serving up fake culture, leeching off the creativity of real human artists." He talks of Artificial Intelligence ofcourse, but also of Algorithms and other factors born from Marketing Strategies. I was at high School and at art class we were going through the esthetics of toilet paper advertisement and the advertisments of washing machines. Usueful products we perceive now, but toilet paper is a commodity that costs money and takes trees and old clothing to be produced due to the need of cellulose. Washing was something that generations of people did using all kinds of implements. The washing machine wasn't needed, so they seduced people in buying them. The side effect was that culturally there was space for habit innovations due to the free time of housewifes, that f.i. now could go work and contribute to inflation and poverty (this is a sarcastic remark), but the washing machine also contributed to an innovation contributed to pollution, extinction of species, and endangering of many more. The story goes that when the water clock was inventyed in China, and it was offered to the emperor as a gift, after some debzting with his courtiers the emperor forbade the broad spread of the clock due to the pressure it would give on time and planning at the expense of the adaptability to natural cycles, such as our internal clockes, the seasons etc. On hindsight, if the story is true or not (the innovation being Chinese is) was on point. Clocktime has become a stresser in life. As such clock time parasites on us. Ted Gioia suggested to "Just take a look at the dominant digital platforms—and consider how little they actually create. But the amount of leeching they do is really quite stunning, especially when compared with the dominant businesses of the past." The tech billionaires have transformed the economic landscape. Many

businesses had to disapear and transform to become digital online stalls in the Amazon marketplace or similar platforms. Earlyer supermarkets took over from the neighbourhood shop, offering more choice, cheaper prices, but also products of significant lesser quality. The sourcing cycle, the production cycle, marketing cycle, selling cycle, life cycle of products, and the 2nd use cycle of products have all been impactful on our lives and have moved us purposefully away from the abiltiy to provide comfort to ourselves. The medical industry has done the same, the political systems likewise created dependencies, and the news cycle and media cycles keep us distracted from life and exited about things that are not in much ways related to us, while witholding to us the promises they have always made on how our lives would become better.

I remember one of my students doing antropological research in Africa, relating to me that he came to a city with a few hundred thousand citizens. There was only electricity for a few hours per day for a few functions, there were hardly anny cars or motorcycles, there was only one muddy road leading there. People went into the fields to collect foods, and people were healthy. But then roads were constructed, the powernetwork established, salaries set, and the differences between poor and rich became established. All of a sudden there were "have and have not's": poverty came, hunger, and disease. Commercial Economy had arrived. It had reduced social and economic mobility and generated inequality on the basis of generating greed.

Diseases linked to economic well-being are sometimes called "diseases of affluence", or noncommunicable diseases (NCDs). They include heart disease, stroke, certain cancers, type 2 diabetes, and chronic respiratory diseases among others. These chonic and deadly diseases are often driven by lifestyle factors like poor diet and physical inactivity that can accompany higher economic status as well as deprivation. Mental health issues and some gastrointestinal diseases can also be associated with economic factors. Our economic progress has made us prone to new diseases, without resolving all of the old ones, (allthough many disease issues have been reduced, f.i. through vaccinations, that admittedly do not work equally good for everyone), But our economic and technological progress has also moved us away from our biological capacity, and has it replaced with for instance romantic ideologies of the body shape, and other facets of our appearance. There is improvement, but not resolvement.

Understanding that progress is not always progress, but can as well be a stap backwards is very important. Zhuangzi, a famous Chinese writer who lived about 2400 years ago, had a meme that said "A weapen is as dangerous as the hand that holds it", that is clearly valuable for much of our innovations. Although the wins of modern society and technology appear amazing, we also lost a lot. The most of what we lost is the freedom to remain autonomous from dependency. That lack of autonomy reduces the validity of political freedom, or the freedom of speech to a large degree.

Because much of what we talk about, in fact is what we complain about: climate change, sports results, quality of food, government policies, salaries, lack of free time, etc. We live live's in servitude, contracted feudal slaves, not quite yet drones, but given technological innovation we might as well get there, and end up in the nightmares of Cyberpunk literature, such as Neil Stephenson's 1992 "Snowcrash", or William Gibson's 1984 "Neuromancer".

So is economic progress than bad? I do not think so, it also helped us to become more aware about the human condition and it's natural a-symmetries. But what I think that does matter is that the economic and technological progression is more like a maze than like a boon. It made us lose sight of much of our humane nature where we are supportive of life and each other, and other beings in a humane way. We are with many, like locusts in the corn field, but like locusts we are also driven to blindly consume due to the addctions and cravings economy has saddled us up with. I believe society needs a change in attitude, namely where economic comfort is balanced with skills of autonomy in the most important fields of our existence: our social relations with fellow people and other beings; our relationship with nourishment and self-improvement; and our relationship with the naturalness of having a relaxed and fit agile body and mind. Just imagine in your place in life, how these three aspects will already change your prospects in career, and patience in dealing with the issues others serve you in life. Personally I think we should make such attitudes compulsory in school education, but also part of training to prepare us for parenting and managing the world and societies at large. What are your ideas about this? I am sure that when you take your time to consider this you are going to agree, and that passively sitting by is not going to help you become autonomous in your health or your role in the world.

From here let us go to the main institute of dependency in relationship to our health: the medical establishments.

Health industry and pollution

Healthcare-based pollution stems from the industry's high consumption of energy, materials, and resources, leading to greenhouse gas emissions, waste generation, and other forms of pollution. This includes emissions from the production of goods, energy use in facilities, transportation, and the disposal of both hazardous and non-hazardous waste, with some estimates placing the sector's contribution to global greenhouse gases at around 5-7%.

The RIVM, a dutch governmental institute has calculated that production of chemical products, including solvents and medicines, accounts for approximately 40% of greenhouse gas emissions. For this reason, the chemical and pharmaceutical industries are responsible for the largest proportion of the healthcare sector's climate footprint.

The World Health Organisation reveals that the total amount of waste generated by health-care activities, about 85% is general, non-hazardous waste. The remaining 15% is considered hazardous material that may be infectious, toxic, carcinogen, flammable, corrosive, reactive, explosive or radioactive. Every year an estimated 16 billion injections are administered worldwide, but not all the needles and syringes are properly disposed of afterwards. Open burning and low-temperature incineration of health care wastes can, under some circumstances, result in the emission of dioxins, furans and particulate matter. From this summary we can see that healthcare is not nescessarily the cleanest industry. But this chapter is not to reveal how vile Modern Healthcare is. Sure it is a main polluting agent with manuy faces, but we pollute much more of the planet and ourselves causing us to need the use of that healthcare. It is our go-to refuge when we start realizing we are damaged goods. But, let me first make clear that I think that many commercial health services do not have our best in mind. Wether it is your neighbourhood holist healer or your academic hospital, or the factory producing anti-cancer medications: financial incentives are going to be part of their 'reason d'etre', their reason for existing. In Chinese medicine there is a saying about doctors that can afford an expensive car: they overcharge their clients. Another saying says that you should treat every client as if it were a family member, so giving discounts is in Chinese medicine morality the core of clinical economy.

I am pretty sure nobody working in healthcare has ill will. Believe me, when you talk with people they have the best intentions, and more often than not they will believe in them, but they are also stakeholders in keeping you as a costumer. And to be fair, if you really make people free of their issues, most of the people feel cheated or distrust you. Many people do not even believe they could be free from the impact of their disease. Mind you, I choose my wording here carefully.

Health does not mean simply mean to be 'without disease', but means being without the negative impact of disease. When a body is properly maintained and developed, many diseases can occur, whithout leading to negative results. I give you one example, namely of a former client. She came with pretty serious complaints, but she did not go to a medical doctor yet. When I made the diagnosis I did so on the basis of Chinese medicine ideas, not on the basis of western medicine diagnosis. I gave her a hefty exercise package to take care of herself, and her symptoms disappeared after a while, so she did well. Every week she came to classes several times and she exercised at home too. For a year or so all went fine. Her life, work, relationship, it all flourished. The disease was in control, but i warned her to keep on exercising all her life to freeze the disease in its tracks. But then she went on a holliday and wanted to celebrate, drank wine, ate ... you know, the stuff people do when on hollidays/ She took no time to keep up her practice. All, her symptoms in a few weeks time recurred, so in a panick she went to see doctor who gave her the diagnosis that she had Multiple Sclerosis, which is a terrible disease. In the years before I worked with a group of patients, all people with this terrible disease. In this group I noticed that many of the clients with progressed disease took a lot of opiate based medication, with side effect muscle cramps, because they said it wouldn't make a difference: they would die anyway. They didn't commit to do exercise because the doctor didn't believe it would do much for them. The diagnosis was like the Sword of Damocles, hanging over their heads, and in fact it diminished their self preservation, and they swallowed in selfishness. I cannot say it nicer, I am sorry if you as a reader suffer MS yourself and take it personal. Just take it as warning and an admonishment to check your own motivations. I certainly do not want to say all MS sufferers will be the same as the people in my group, but what i say is that if the determination by western diagnosis is made, it is hard to escape a growing fatalist trust in the diagnosis' predictiove quality. Because also many of these clients were smart enough to understand what was going on, but they gamed their unavoidable end results. They were sitting life out, so to say.

Their biggest problem was in fact the diagnosis that said the end result was unavoidable. So for the one client I mentioned I avoided the diagnosis, so that could experience for herself the power that she had over her disease. The likelyhood that it would make the disease go away was small, but it definately increased her survivability if she did not have the death sentence that the medical diagnosis was. This and many stories like this keep bothering my heart ever since. I do not want to demote the validity of modern medical science and achievement, but I also like to emphasise its relative ignorance, and its authoritatian control over our lives. Let's get a bit deeper on this subject.

In a larger scope we see that our medical systems are generally focussed on crisis management. In an article on "Crisis Pricing"

John F. Duffy and Richard M. Hynes wrote that: "Emergencies happen. By definition, they are exceptional; they create uncertainty; they cause disruption; and they often lead to massive adjustments and changes within society. In law too, crisis and emergency pose deep challenges and often demand significant adjustments. Perhaps because this young century has already seen its share of crises—a coordinated terrorist attack, a great recession, a global pandemic, and a large ground war in Europe—an exceptionally large literature has developed around the questions whether, and to what extent, crises should lead the law to sacrifice or at least suspend rules applicable in ordinary times." he also explain that the economic literature on market crises parallels the literature on law in times of crisis to an extraordinary degree. They show that like in the legal literature, the economic environment also has rights. They explain there is a business-as-usual moniker that is at least as apt in describing the market libertarian position, for it literally supports continuing business as in usual times. In other words, the proper regulatory response is to stay the course—to allow markets to function without any special governmental intervention. Regulatory literature includes a market libertarian, business-as-usual position that closely parallels the civil libertarian approach to constitutional structures. Over time markets have become liberalized to give them free reign to shape the market with disruption and innovation. When things go awry, governments will likely buy them out so they can easily restart. The problem here to note is that Healthcare and crisis management as a result have become more and more a libertarian business concept, and less a purpose of providing health and care to everyone. Health has in many cases a price tag, and that price tag in fact contributes to the pending world crisis we see so many signs of in the news nowadays. Healthcare is offered as a product, and we as people with health needs can only look at the price and judge if their solution is worth the economic suffering or not. Some escape is possible, namely by paying forward on health risks through an insurance. Basically you pay forward on a potential need that you have, that they use to invest in the stockmarket, buildings, space industry, pharmaceutical industry, or even weapons. That health supportive price tag in some countries is so high that it can absorb much of people's income to just hang on, let alone to find a good solution. Or they have to abandon all hope and just sit out their disease or trauma. The healthcare industry has generated an autoritorian control over our health, suggesting freedom of choice, while in fact milking our financial capacity, while when our money is drained, letting us dry out in the cold. Siure statistically they help people and take their value from their successes. The statistical successes do not say anything over the people excluded from entry into the system, or had to prematurely exit it.

We might think, like in the EU, that market forces are guided by government regulations, but these are revolving around the rights of companies as much as in, say, the USA. In fact, around the world there are recognitions for human rights on health. The most of the countries are signatories of these rights, although not all countries have funds to provide for that health. UN and Unesco funds are continuously directed to the poorest areas of the world to provide a bare minimum of food, housing and healthcare. I started working with Rohingya refugees, probably inspired by the fact that they heard about this project and they asked me to help them use this project to provide them with healthcare they can manage themselves. Other factors were refugee camp with Tibetan refugeess I visited in the past when residing in Nepal. Many lived in tents in deplorable poverty, guarded by Nepali Police and UN forces. I was in Bosnia after the war there was just finished, and I could close up witness the victims of the war: people, buildings, infrastructure. Seeing refugees travel from Asia in Boats to Australia, or from North-Africa, Central Asia, and supporting defensive care here in my local region.

I was shocked how much people nowadays protest the arrival of refugees. It is noted that it splits families apart. My own sister doesnt talk to me because I asked her to tone down on the baseless accusations of forreigners to be guilty of about everything wrong in the coiuntry, while she very well knows her sister in law is forreign and her nieces are likewise at risk. There is no awarenes of the fact that they themselves can become refugees and that what now happens to refugees might happen to them. People seem to see refugees as a lawless bunch and fortune seekers, while in fact in most cases crisis areas gradually develop. And people develop new habits to adapt, untill it becomes unbearable. Becoming a refugee is usually the last people plan.

The UNHRC (Hunited Nations Human Rights Council) shows on their information page that Refugees are people forced to flee their own country and seek safety in another country. They are unable to return to their own country because of feared persecution as a result of who they are, what they believe in or say, or because of armed conflict, violence or serious public disorder.

Nowadays Climate disaster is more and more often a reason to flee home. There are many reasons for poverty, so looking for greener pastures is a factor too.

Many have been forced to flee with little more than the clothes on their back, leaving behind their homes, possessions, jobs and loved ones, but not their bad memories. They may have suffered human rights violations, being injured in their flight, or seen family members or friends killed or attacked.

There were 42.7 million refugees globally at the end of 2024, the most recent reporting period. UNHRC, the UN Refugee Agency, is mandated to protect 31 million refugees and 5.9 million other people in need of international protection. A further 5.9 million Palestine refugees are supported by the United Nations Relief and Works Agency for Palestine Refugees in the Near East (UNRWA), which was set up in 1949 to care for displaced Palestinians. Non of any of these people was prepared for such a situation. That is pretty much a drama , isn't it? If people are not moved by that drama there is something very wrong with them. They lack the kindness that is natural to people, and they might have already got so much fear for life in them that the mere touch of problems already gets them into the defense. I hope this book can help these people to find their humanity by helping them consider that they might also be at risk. I think our modern society has great education if it wants to, especially on the technical and economic front, but in understanding health and developing a bit of altruism would have definately been more helpful.

The The Joint Research Centre, the EU Science Hub from the European Counsel states that "Around 87 million Europeans are exposed to multiple natural hazards". A first-time assessment at the level of local administrative units shows nearly 19% of Europe's population is exposed to multiple natural hazards. Beyond population density, the income level is the primary driver that influences risk status. They analysed data on six hazards: coastal flooding, river flooding, landslides, earthquakes, wildfires, and soil shrinking and swelling (subsidence), on the basis of population and economic information. There is a paper in which they mapped out the local administrative units (municipalities or communes) most exposed to multiple hazards.

Disasters are sometimes considered externa shocks, but disaster risk results from the complex interaction between development processes that generate conditions of exposure, vulnerability and hazard. Disaster risk is therefore considered as the combination of the severity and frequency of a hazard, the numbers of people and assets exposed to the hazard, and their vulnerability to damage. A share of 21.4% of local administrative units in the EU27 and the UK, home to approximately 87 million people, are exposed to multiple hazards. Nearly half of this population (about 40 million people) faces exposure to three or more hazards. In France, the highest number of local administrative units is exposed (around 7000; although it also has the largest number of municipalities), followed by Italy, Slovenia, Bulgaria, Spain, Germany and Romania, the latter counting around 1000 municipalities exposed. In terms of population, Italy has the highest number of people exposed to multiple hazards, with 21.4 million residents exposed. Together with the Netherlands, France, Spain, and Germany, these five countries account for 55% of the EU's population exposed to multi-hazards. That is scary. For me living in a city 6 meters under sea level it feels quite normal. In the past I actually rarely thought about it. I trusted that the government would take precautions, as the country has experienced disastous flooding frequently. But in fact due to conservative and liberal politics costs of maintenance and development has skyrocketed and people have moved projects forward. On top of that we see chemicals, microplastics and airpollution, new diseases and other issues we get to discuss later becoming new disaster factors. Hing Keung Ma wrote in a 2017 article named:" The Development of Altruism with Special Reference to Human Relationships"[xiii], he stated that human relationships involve some form of cost and benefit calculations, and together with altruism this forms the foundation upon which human relationships are built. In his thought I think he creates a feedback system between opportunity thinking and compassionate interaction, although he doesn't say that explicitly. He proposed a Taxonomy of Altruism. He saw the positioning between altruism and opportunism as a sliding scale. He classified human relationships into three major groups: "primary group, secondary group, and tertiary group. The primary group consists of members that are very closely related to each other either by genetic relatedness (e.g., parents, siblings, and cousins) or social relatedness (e.g., mate and close friends) or both. Altruism comes more easy to close family or community members. The secondary group consists of members that are socially related but also less closely related with each other (e.g., people of the same political or religious group, teachers, mentors, acquaintances, neighbors, working colleagues, and strangers). Here the urge to act inclusive already is much smaller. Lastly, the tertiary group consists of members of other species (e.g. pets, cattle, wild animals, birds). Here the altruist impuls for many is almost not there, that is why they can be fervent eaters of meat. Some have much altruism for animals and nature, sometimes due to trauma with people. But still most combine care for animals with eating meat, fish or both. A religious group like the Jains in India and Pakistan abhor from causing suffering for any living creature. But also in the west more and more people choose vegetarianism, even if only for ecological reasons.

Hing Keung Ma describes two developmental principles of altruism. The first principle states that the development of altruism follows the 10-stage theory and moves from Stage 1: Egoism, toward the higher stages of altruism slowly. His second developmental principle states that the taxonomy of human relationships is valid at any stage of altruism development. In other words, people at any stage of altruism are more altruistic toward their kin and mate, and then close friends, extended family members, and so on. They are least altruistic toward enemies and members of non-human species. What would be nice, is if the education of extending one's altruism to all species would be part of normal life and child education. Do you agree with me? I think Altruism should also be at the core of any healthcare organisation, and then perhaps capitalisation, leaning on pricing and profits will disappear.

If you do not agree with me and you belief in Darwin's survival of the fittest, or Richard Dawkin's Selfish Gene, let me then tell you a piece of a conversation I once had with Tibetan Lama Rimpochee I was studying Death Rituals and Bardo Teachings with in Bodinath, Nepal. He was speaking with me on "Good" and "Evil". So read along and follow me into the realm of Moral Relativism.

Let me first explain the ideas of Moral Relativism. It is more important than most people are aware of. Our society is sort of build on the idea. Moral relativism is the view that moral judgments are true or false only relative to some particular standpoint, for instance, that of a culture or a historical period, and that no standpoint is uniquely privileged over all others. Chinese medicine for instance is seen as valuable in relationship to ancient Chinese culture, but nowadays we have modern science so than these methods are not enough relevant anymore. From a moral relativist perspective, this appreciation highlights how knowledge systems and practices are shaped by cultural heritage and historical context. Different cultures may uphold varied medical practices as morally and socially valid based on their own traditions and beliefs. Thus, within the context of ancient Chinese culture, traditional medicine holds significant value and meaning. But in a modern context that might not be so. The acknowledgment of modern science introduces a contrasting value system. Moral relativism posits that what is considered "relevant" or "valid" can change over time and across cultural contexts. In contemporary society, medical practices may be viewed through the lens of scientific rigor and empirical evidence. This reflects a shift in values rather than an absolute devaluation of traditional methods. What we can say is that modern science relies on empirical data and experimentation, traditional Chinese medicine draws on centuries of experiential knowledge and cultural practices. Each has its own "truth" based on the cultural frameworks that shape them. Hence, from a moral relativistic viewpoint, one set of methods is not inherently more legitimate than the other; rather, their value is intertwined.

Let me now return to the story of the Tibetan Lama I was talking with. This Lama Rimpchee, who's name has gotten lost in my memories, asked me about someone's actions if they were morally good or evil. It was about a more or less shady Lama who I and some of my friends thought was of questionable behavior. The Lama Rimpochee, let us call him LR, asked me what is "Goodness". I must say that answering that question was not easy. LR said that no matter how much good you try to do, there will be negative effects of what you do, so that there will be victims of your goodness. He said that goodness is an intention, but one that never can result in 100% good results. If your intention is selfish or even evil, likewise, "Evil" actions might have surprizing constructive side effects. In general people like to see as evil self-defeating, because people will eventually turn against you and punish you for your actions. But if that happens, LR suggested, you are not truly evil, you just didn't think it through properly. LR suggested that true evil would include actions of goodness to help avoid people turning against you. That total evil includes calculated acts of goodness to be able to live long and perform the evil you like to perform. LR suggested that neither Pure Evil, nor Pure Goodness is common, rare in fact, because such inclusive thinking is hard to develop. LR also said that both aiming for pure goodness and pure evil lead to enlightenment, a big idea of Buddhism, which in itself is hard to explain. Enlightenment represents a state of profound spiritual awakening and freedom from the cycle of suffering and rebirth called samsara. It is achieved by gaining a deep understanding of the true nature of reality, which involves realizing that all phenomena are impermanent and selfless. Translated that means that the universe isn't personal in its relationship to you. In Daoism that is worded by Laozi in a similar way by stating that "Heaven treats people like straw toys" in The Daodejing (= weft of morality). Key aspects include extinguishing negative states like anger, greed, delusion, and as a result to reach a state of inner peace called nirvana, while developing infinite compassion for all beings. Buddhist enlightenment we can say therefore intents to choose for goodness over evil. Outside the purity of all actions we can say there are going to be relativistic outcomes we cannot control. Being aware of altruist tendencies in ourselves, helps us direct ourself towards Goodness, and prevent being evil or ambigious in our life's choices, at least when we make the choice to do so. Being ambiguous means that we simply do not care enough about the outcomes. Modern healthcare isn't good or evil. It is ambiguous, so what it does, either good or evil is accidental to the process. An economic calculation is made of costs versus benefits. Ambiguity is sort of an indifference isn't it? Relativism is more inclusive.

What I like to conclude this chapter with is that Modern healthcare is focussed more on economy than on helping people on the one side, and secondly that they are to dependent on product based and technology based methodologies. As a result of that the risk is there that in times of crisis as a system it is ill prepared and might collaps under pressures at the expense of clients.

In: "Understanding the Effect of Economic Recession on Healthcare Services: A Systematic Review"[xiv] in the Iranian Journal of Public Health (2022), Raquel Sánchez Recio, Juan Pablo Alonso Pérez De Ágreda, María José Rabanaque, and Isabel Aguilar Palacio wrote that: "Of 3,685 studies, ... regarding 'Effects of the social structure' healthcare accessibility inequalities increased by socioeconomic levels, especially in unemployed, people with low educational levels and migrants. Regarding 'Healthcare effect', the impact of the recession was observed in unmet needs, pharmaceutical spending containment, reduction of hospital beds, and privatization of services". On financial disaster for hosptitals they found that some authors have reported a reduction in the number of hospital beds to contain health expenditure. In Spain, closure of wards has been observed together with the reduction of hospital beds. This situation, along with changing inclusion criteria for waiting lists, is leading to an increase in waiting time for patients. Private Clinic (PC) physicians had greater difficulty in referring patients for Surgical Clinics (SC), or that waiting times had been significantly increased. The impact of the increased waiting time varied among autonomous regions due to the different policies applied. The Irish government observed increased pressure on the provision of hospital beds following the economic crisis-related cuts. A reduction in beds would need to be compensated by adequate investment in public health infrastructure, health promotion and PC services.

In this article The most common reason for an unmet medical need in 2012 was the cost of medical care (36%), followed by waiting lists (15%) (50). Non-EU migrants had the highest prevalence of enforced unmet needs in the majority of countries, with the exception of Spain and Portugal (20). In Spain, only undocumented migrants had problems. In Italy, migrants reported a significant increase in needs compared to the indigenous population since the onset of the economic crisis. Likewise, in Europe, people in lower social classes have six times more unmet needs than people from higher classes in society. I guess we are still living in a class conscious society, or because many people are not in the know about these things, in a class-unconcious society.

I only took a few references from the article as an example, but my point is to point out how fragile a profit based healthcare is, and that just like with a paid parking system that doesn't solve parking problems, insurances do not resolve healthcare needs, nor is the so called competetive free market. It is the high costs in healthcare for the people in need that does. That can put healthcare out of business. They invented the word "affordability" for that. It is something on the edge of what is too much so that users are gradually drained of the funds to hang on. Let alone what can happen when disaster of more serious kinds strikes. Most people will be without healthcare for prolonged amounts of time. Being a refugee leaves it in the hands of those we didn't treat well ourselves to help us. There is a chance they will close their borders for us and lock us into concentrationcamps in the region where we come from. You might recognize that ideology from the news in your country. If people like you and me have not learned to prepare for such risks in life, the disaster only arrives with more problems than was actually needed. So how can we help ourselves? It is clear that from industrial medicine we will only get more of the same, if anything. They might turn top the language of natural and holistic, but they will still root in sales and dependency programming. We cannot do totally without indiustrial medicine. They can do things that natural medicine might not be able to reach on short term. But it is in what can be achieved on an individual basis, and as a community through pro-active learning. What can be summarized from this chapter is thaty there are two kinds of pollution we can talk of: 1) there is the material pollution of the world, and there is 2) the moral pollution of the world.

Holism

Holism is the principle that the identities of objects and events derive from the relational context in which they are embedded. In East Asian Thought systems like Buddhism and Daoism that is described as 'interdependent existence". Reality is seen as a mesh, a 经-Jing, the word that is used for books that describe the interconnectedness between forms and functions. It is a form of causality theory. It means that nothing can happen without having an extended influence on the rest of existence. Buddhism sees it purpously influencing of the trajectory of reality, or history as "moving the 8 spoked wheel of Karma. Karma is a causality theory, mostly referring to moral implications of our actions and that shape history. But the Karma of mountains is to protect landscapes from hot or cold weather, although it is likely not on purpose. So usually we use Karma in situations that required a decission. Holism is more appropriate for the larger schope of Karma. In Daoism we swpeak of Taiji and Yinyang theory to describe the karma and interconnectedness between everything. The Yijing is its explanatory diagram. The text isn't. The so called ten wings try to explain it.

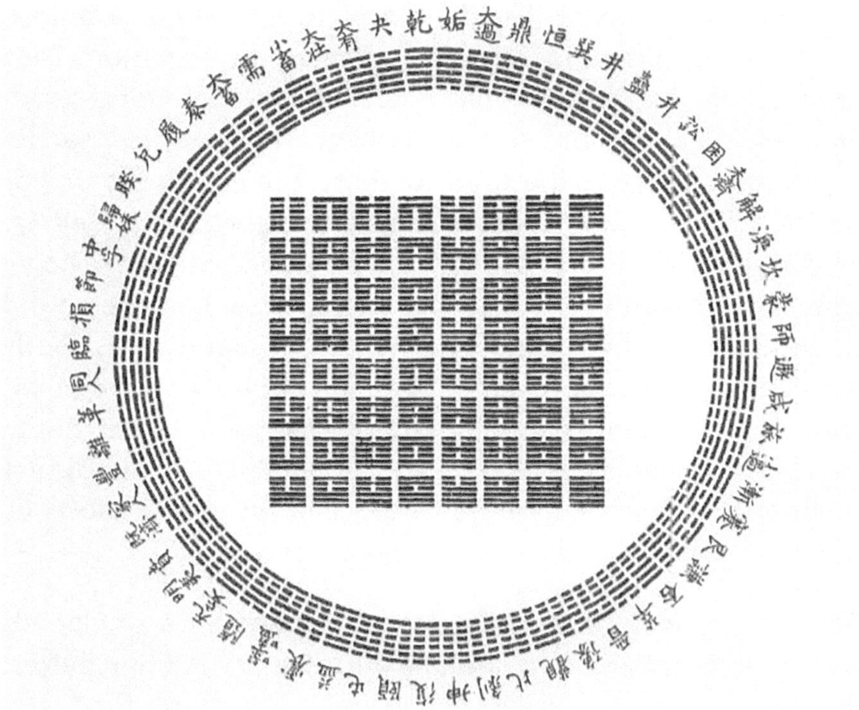

[yijing map of heaven and earth]

Like in the Yijing (Yi= exchange, Jing=weft) in Holism we say that "wholes define parts and parts define wholes". The classic example is the relation of components of a sentence. Patterns of letters form words and particular organizations of words form sentences. Clearly, the meaning of the sentence depends on its individual words (parts define whole). At the same time, the meaning of words is often defined by the meaning of the sentence (wholes define parts). In both Buddhism and Daoism the body is seen as a wholist whole and that holism is described in different fashion.

For instance we can recognize ourselves as human both through our human form and our moral compas. I feed the crows in my street nearly every day. When I forget they call out to me to help me remember, or they demonstratively go sit on a lantern pole in front of my house trying to catch my attention. They understand I feel morally obliged to maintain my feeding habit. They are a couple, but the one collects most of the peanuts I give them without the urge to share them with his or her partner. They do not have that same moral guilt about feeding. Hing keung Ma's Altruism theory I explained above is providing a moral framework for our actions. If we care we can be moved to act. In our body we see we can cut things out of our body without stopping the feeling to be human. But we haven't yet gone so far as to investigate how far we can go with that. But in the theory of interdependence we can see that every bodypart contributes something to the whole, and the whole allows us to let the bodyparts do specific things.

Daoism sees Holism and interdependence as a starting point. We can self-cultivate and finetune ourselves to function better. We can do this in the knowledge field, the moral field, the skill field and the biological functions field, just to name a few. This book's second part is letting you practice some of these skills to improve the general wellbeing of your body. On that is the content of the research we later go discuss build. The knowledge is ages old, but mostly forgotten due to the emphasis on modern scientific explanation. Modern science is continuously rediscovering things from other cultures, is deconstructing them and rebuilding it in its own way. It makes me sometimes think about a cartoon I used to read as a child: someone was taking a mechanical alarmclock apart because it was broken. After repairing it by re-ensambling it it would indeed work, but there would always be a few parts left that the character couldnt place, or there were some parts missing, so he had to improvise to make it work. Holist mesh theory sees the missing parts causing problems over time. The ecological movement is based on that idea: we took out some elements from nature so that we -like locusts- could increase our numbers exponentially and overrun other species, and exploit nature to a degree that gave me this laptop to write this book for you, and to design my research to try to contribute something ancient to the future, in the hope of repairing it a bit together with you and your imput, however late we are in the process.

Within the hardcore ideas of ecological idealism we as a species are out of control, we are more like a disease than a blessing, however we as individuals might think about that. But we are here and are not consciously suicidal, certainly not on an individual basis. So what we need to learn is how to restore some form of natural balance and harmonious co-existence so that nature can restore and refind its natural interdependency by developing a new weft (Jing, remember?). That will take tens of thousands of years. It might even spark a new evolutionary boom.

Holism is a great thought, but holism isn't really easy to encapsulate in scientific concepts. As a theory it can accept it, I think, but comprehending it might be more difficult. Holist systems are mostly organic in nature. For scientific thought, theories are described as either localizationist or holist. Localizationist theories are the bulk of exploration. It describes every thing as an independent unit, much as our property laws allow us to own a piece of the world or have country borders. A chair is a chair, and a table is a table. These theories are quite narrow in scope. Unlike localizationist theories, science and scientific philosophy think that there is no one holist model that has emerged as the major example of this class of theories. However, several lines of evidence are adduced as evidence for holist theories, and all holist theories suffer from similar inadequacies in accounting for certain empirical findings within their usual reductive ways of thinking. By nature a holist something cannot be described by its parts, and thus have they come up with emergent theories. The ideas about AI are like that. Modern science sees consciousness as an emergent property from the constellation of Chemicals in our body. It has difficulty in describing what being alive means other than an emergent property. On top of that emergence consciousness also emerges. It is a piramid of emergent properties that are neither things not not there.

Holism is often explained as emergent systems, but from the Chinese Daoist perspective holism is the acceptance of the `thisness' and , nowness' of reality, where this-ness and now-ness are self generating continuous properties, that are embedded in both change and continuous existence. Does this clarify the idea of interdependent existence? In fact it declares that reality is a paradox that doesn't have a cause to exist nor to not exist. Some resolve that paradoxicality by placing a divine being as the creater of reality. That does seem to help but puts the paradox only behind the divine being. So what daoist holism does, is accept the reality we live in, and try to put it to our hands by using nature, not by going with the flow and not by going against it and taking it apart.

Going with the flow is seen as a sign of lack of consciousness, much like a branch floating on a river. The willingness to take it apart and think we know better than nature is also seen as a lack of conciousness. Learning to become conscious beings is at the core of using nature to improve life and ourselves.

To do so we do not need complex machines to do our observations for us, we also do not need tools to do our calculations for us. We need to develop a feel for life and learn to measure by observation and recognize the harmony that allows us to live in the Jing/mesh without experiencing resistance. I do not think there is a better word to describe health and healthy lifestyle.

The language of such a lifestyle represents experience, it is emperical, and not technological. The theories of Daoism and Chinese medicine use such language. It describes the experiences of being and disease in simple environmental concepts, such as warm, cold, dampy, windy, open, close, decrepit, oppulent, neutral, fast slow, hard, soft etc. etc. Things that are immedeately clear to us when we experience them. They are at the root of the vocabulary we learned to recognize as a child. Children have not got a grasp of reality yet, but over time due to movement, observation, talking and experiencing they build a holist experience of life. At school they are made aware of how to dissect things and take a reductionist and localizationist view on life. These views are the same. Reductionism tries to bring things back to their smallest component. It is what makes nano technology and computer chips possible. A robot is a reductionist person. There is no embodyment of consciousness in a robot.

Embodyment is seen as a complex dynamical system in the behavioral sciences. It means that cognition and action arise from interactions between brain, body and the environment . The social scientists Thelen, Shoner, Scheier and Schmidt did coauthor a paper on that in 2001. Spencer et al. Reflected on that in 2006, and they concluded that as a result, perception, action, and cognition form an integrated system that cannot be partitioned. They see that 'Embodiment' is a specific form of the more general theoretical stance of 'holism'. Here, holism refers to how any system relates to its parts and assumes non-reducibility, explained as properties of the system that cannot be reduced to properties of its parts. But Holism also refers here to non-separability, where parts of the system cannot be separated from the system as a whole. This was best summarized by Lundh in 2015. Combined with the phenomena of soft-assembly and co-regulation, a complex dynamical systems approach fits within the 'holistic-interactionistic paradigm' as defined by Magnusson in 2001. It also fits with the current shift in social cognition research, which moves away from their traditional focus on the individual's capacities towards an embodied and participatory view of social understanding. Social intelligence.

All in all we have now discussed holism in a variety of ways, namely as a meshed reality, as non- reductability and non-seperability, as embodyment, as interdependent existence, and as having need for its own experience based language. This book is written from the experience of the non separation between heart and behaviour, mind and body, self and environment, environment and behaviour and self and health. In general nowadays we see holism as a part of Natural medicine. Let us now investigate a bit in natural medicine systems.

Natural medicines and Holism

In general Natural Medicine, also known as naturopathy, is seen as a system of healthcare that uses natural therapies to help the body heal itself. It takes a holistic approach, focusing on prevention and addressing the root cause of disease through methods like diet, exercise, stress management, herbs, and other supplements. As you can see based on the previous chapter the approach to that definition still is localizationist in outlook. It does focus on the thingness of the body, and doesn't meet the seemless integration of the being with the world. We can call this limited holism "exclusionist holism", It still is based on the individual human unit.

There are some key understandings we need to take into account when discussing natural therapies. A natural therapist will say that he or she will identify and treat the cause to focus on finding and addressing the root cause of an illness, but as we have seen above, it is often the social or climatic environment that casues our health problems. And as a therapist you cannot do much about that. Saying it is the fault of the kidney, or a spirit, or a particular enzyme, it is akin to saying: "It is your own fault". Therefore although it is good to understand the internal workings of a body, it will never be sufficient to adress root causes. Disease is as much -if not more- a social issue as it is a biological issue owned by the person. Adressing the root cause means adressing the social, educational and power systems of the world. In the past we would have said that the external factor is a possessing being, be it ghost, spirit, demon, shaitan, virus, fungus, or bacteria. In TCM we often say that disharmony of the interior creates the climatic environment that allows external climatic factors to aggravate the internal disturbances. This is an interaction between the interior and the exterior environments, Meaning that Disease is a negotiated factor. Modern TCM actually puts the cause of the issue in the human unit. It sees the self as a soldier that has to defend against the exterior. In Daoism they used to speak of reaching inner coordination, enlightenment, and inner peace in such a way that external forces did not feel like attacking us.

They called this Taiyi-太乙, 'bigger unity', the unity between ourself and the world at large. Daoists call this 'becoming everlasting like Heaven and Earth', Immortality in fact.

Natural Therapies often invoke the healing power of nature, which is to support the body's inherent ability to heal itself. The reality is that self healing means healing induced by the body itself, a concept borrowed from immunology. Immunology discusses functional resistance against disease factors. Immunity to a disease is achieved through the presence of antibodies to that disease in a person's system. There are two types of immunity: active and passive. Active immunity is triggered by a disease making factor, such as a virus. Immunity in that sense is naturally there or vaccin induced. Many diseases we have no resistance for, and becasue of that many vaccins are developed as artificial development for immunity. Passive immunity is also artificially induced, namely by injecting ready made antibodies into somebody.

From the Daoland perspective, the body is a creature of habit: it aims to restore normalcy. We have a range of glands that work on that. These habits can be destructive, such as walking in a slanted position, drinking alcohol, smoking, eating too much etc. In spite of all these bad habits, when we try to change them we run into problems due to the self-restoritative capacity of the body. That is self healing pur sang. The body understands habit in the context of organisation.

Science often speaks of the intelligence of the forming of the body as if coming from the Genes, but when the body is there our habits alter these genes. In Chinese medicine we see the self restorativeness as a function of the kidneys. In TCM immunity is seen as a function of the 卫/衛氣 Weiqi, originating in the lungs but made from the recombination of 空氣 Kongqi and 骨氣 Guqi, 'functional emptiness', and the 'essence of grains'. Weiqi is a Chinese board game of territory conquering and guarding. Wei means guarding, but then because of the function in the body it also means reaching out and conquering. In fact in The huangdineijing Weiqi is seen as an envoy of sorts. It carries the message of the emperor to places in the body that need orders. The weiqi envoy races on the back of a horse (metaphorically), which is made of the blood, stored in the stables of the liver (also metaphorically). The blood also doubles as soldiers, and as workers. Weiqi is therefore not the defense itself, but the messenger that has to correct situations by transporting orders. The weiqi doesn't do anything itself. It is the totality of the whole body and self being coordinated that makes the body impervious to external influence. But what we do learn from this is that this whole has to have an active, even a bit wild lifestyle to generate internally activity to maintain wholeness. There was not really an idea of immunity in Chinese Medicine. It is one of these ideas we mentioned above as western influence that in medicine entered China via Japan.

There was an idea of broken harmony. This idea was based on ideas of civilization and wilderness. The city was civilization, and the countryside was wilderness. Wilderness still had order. But everything beyon that, such as described in the Chinese Han dynasty text "Shanghaijing", 'weft of mountains and seas', it talks of the areas beyond the order where ghosts, demons and other monsters live. Our body has to be seen as a similar construction. The main organs are the civil cities or palaces, and the remainder of the body is the wilderness. What is beyon the body listens to a different order of which little can be understoon or seen, unless when we do not keep ourselves ordered, we become part of that world outside ourselves, in that the world and us blend into each other, which in modern terms would probably be akin to a dissociation or dissolving process. This process is called 虛 Xü-decrepicy. Decrepicy is the kind of weakness of decrepit construction. It means the Jing (our act of cohering ourselves) is weak, we are not good at holding ourselves together. It is one of the core concerns in the history of Chinese medicine: how do we secure the Jing. The Jing allows for sort of a hermetic holism. If something is hermetic it is a system sort of closed onto itself. It doesn't decay and therefore is eternal. Our activities in life depend on that and if the jing degrades we age and get sick. Unlike in western medicine -as I explain elsewhere in the book as well, Jing is not build on a substance we have, but is based on body memory (the yinjing) and the body cohering (the yangjing). In yin yang theory we say that yin generates yang and yang feeds yin. Now you know how repetetive acting in exercise helps you to grow better in a particular action.

But peculiar in modern ideas of holism is that it seems quite egalitarian, or diffuse even. Chinese holism is hierarchical. Although it is holist, it internal polarity (taiji) also generates hierarchies.

These hierarchies are established through the separation of things in combinations of yin and yang as opposites that also become each other, and are therefore fluid in quality. They represent the workings of a country, or a citystate of central civility and the surrounding countryside/landscape. The yinjing and yangjing system as described above is such a fluid system. The Wuxing system of five manifest forms of consuming (water-like, wood-like, fire-like, earth-like, and metal-like) is more organic and asymetrical. It introduces life in reality. Wuxing therefore only applies to living systems. Handling wuxing systems are therefore in Daoism and Confucianism seen as moral systems. When one of them goes outside its range or retreats, it causes damage. All of them have yin and yang aspects, starting with jing, then self awareness (shen), and increased effectiveness, eventually becoming self evident action (qi)

In environmentalism there is a discussion about the validation of environmental holism, and environmental individualism. I hope you understand where I go to with this: environmental holism is about the holeness of the environment and how it maintains itself. Environmental individualism discusses the rights in how individual animal can manifest itself as it pleases. Our human nature puts us ofcourse in the latter category. Abby Matt wrote and article for Indiana University's 'Religious studies undergraduate journal' (2016). She argues for Hierarchical Holism as a means to combine holist and the individualist view in an ethics aiming for soft boundaries. She borrowed the concept from 'Individualism, Holism, and Environmental Ethics', written by Kristin Shrader- Frechette, and published in "The Environment in Anthropology: A Reader in Ecology, Culture, and Sustainable Living" edited by Nora Haenn and Richard R. Wilk in 2006. She summarizes hierarchical holism as such: "We might call this integrated position "hierarchical holism" because it recognizes the plausibility of attributing inherent worth (therefore the status of moral patients) to systems and processes that are not sentient, yet it provides for a hierarchical or lexicographic ordering of various duties regarding humans, other beings, and environmental systems or processes". She divides hierarchical holism in 3 prominent characteristics:

- (1) *it is based on a metaphysical rather than merely a scientific notion of nature as a community;*
- *(2) it relies on an ethics that sees people as the center of the world, but also life in a larger sense*
- *(3) it includes second-order moral principles capable of adjudicating conflicts among human versus nonhuman interests.*

I think this is similar to the altruist stages discussed earlyer. It also shows that holism is a much more complicated issue than is being discussed in popular discussions on holism. Holism is not a simple physics based manifestation of everything relating to everything else, but it is also a moral approach to reality and health/healthcare, and it puts us in a two-fold relationship with nature: self-centered and merged with nature as a whole. When we exercise, or are in the process of healing or self-healing, we depend on both what nature has to offer us and in how we contribute to nature. Holism then can be seen as a two way street. It gives us something, and we equally have to give us back. The problem now is modern naturapath therapies.

What we see from most natural medicine systems is that they aren't holistic. They are a combination of physics based biology and environmental individualism. The naturopath perspective sees the right for the individual to use nature for itself, and it supports this by means of the mechanisms of modern biochemistry. We might finance the green movement or do other supportive acts, but it is nothing compared to what we do not do to give back. We do not become more part of nature.

When we seek out natural therapies, a core aspect natural therapies talk about is that they are environment friendly. The production process of items aims to use the least invasive and most natural process in factories. The same goes to the approach in the use of natural therapies.

Another aspect is the treatment of the whole person. In natural therapies there is the consideration of the patient's overall health, including physical, mental, and emotional factors. Another aspect is that of disease prevention in naturopath approaches, which emphasizes preventing disease and promoting health before anything serious can happen. Our project is especially focussed on that, but it also wants to point out that specific, more animist and hierchical holist approach of embedding onself in nature to develop health. Chinese medicine has always played around wioth the moral dimensions of health and disease. In the Huangdineijing from 2600 years ago in the first chapters it says that Jing is broken down by desires, anger and fear. They force us on a path of self fulfilment, creating disharmony with nature at large. The problem for most people ofcourse is that we see anger, desire and fear not nescessarily as either good or bad, becasue we feel most of these feelings, which we see as negative are usually relative mild feelings of desire, fear and anger. Chinese medicine on the other hand, suggests that all individually bound emotions, such as joy (happiness and love), anger, worry, grief, fear, fright, and contemplation/pensiveness) are constructs rooted in anger, fear and desire. They see that these three are expressions of "aversion", while the only animist and altruist feeling we need for health is "affinity". In affinity we are capable to connect with all living systems. With aversion we turn ourselves away from connectivity. It is this disconnection that causes disharmony, which in turn is cause for the formation of disease. . From here I think it is interesting to have a look at tribal medicine systems.

Tribal medicine systems

Modern biochemical medicine often looks at plant-based solutions in other cultures for generating its medications. There is an irony in that, because traditional medicine systems are frowned upon as a healing modality. But let me give you 3 examples the World Health Organization offers.

1) After testing over 240 000 compounds for use in antimalarial medicals, Chinese scientist Tu Youyou, head of the Project 523 to discover a cure for chloroquine-resistant malaria, turned to traditional Chinese medical literature for clues. There, she and her team found a reference to sweet wormwood to treat intermittent fevers. In 1971, Tu Youyou's team isolated artemisinin, an active compound in sweet wormwood that was particularly effective in treating malaria. They didn't

recognize that likely more compounds in the artemisia jointly were responsib;le for the effect of Chinese herbal solutions. But Artemisinin is now recommended by the World Health Organization as the first and second line of treatment for malaria. In 2015, Tu Youyou was awarded the Nobel Prize in Physiology or Medicine for her work on malaria, which has saved millions of lives. Would it have been possible to reach the same goal by using Artemisia itself?

In a 2013 article Julia Mouton, Olivia Jansen, Michel Frédérich, Frank van der Kooy co-authored an article to investicate artemisia tea effect on malaria compared to Artemisinin as a pure compound, to see if the compound substace synergy of the plant would perform better or worse than the extract. What they found is that the effect was more or less the same. Growing the plant locally for tea medicine then would have been as effective and more cheap than building factories to extract and package the medication.

2) Willow bark as the basis of aspirin is another example of how nature and traditional knowledge have contributed to modern medicine. From over 3500 years ago, bark from the willow tree was used as a pain reliever and an anti-inflammatory by Sumerians and Egyptians. In later years, it was used to ease the pain of childbirth in ancient Greece and cure fevers. In the 1897, Bayer chemist Felix Hoffmann synthesized aspirin and the drug has gone on to improve, and save, the lives of millions of people every day – with multiple benefits including preventing heart attack or stroke, improving blood pressure, and relieving pain and swelling. Aspirin is now one of the most used drugs in the world.

Many believe that willow is the natural source of aspirin. However, willow species contain only a low quantity of the prodrug salicin which is metabolized during absorption into various salicylate derivatives. Asperin is a high concentration dosage, comparable with how Chinese herbal medicine makes herbal soups to extract more of the aromatic oils. But in Willow bark salicin isn't the only relevant substance. For willow bark, also flavonoids and polyphenols contribute to the potent willow bark analgesic and anti-inflammatory effect. The multi-component active principle of willow bark provides a broader mechanism of action than aspirin and is devoid of serious adverse events. In contrast to synthetic aspirin, willow bark does not damage the gastrointestinal mucosa.

3) The Madagascar periwinkle, which is the source of childhood cancer drugs vinblastine and vincristine has an exceptionally long history of being used as a medicinal plant, and finds mention in Mesopotamian folklore, the Ayurveda system of traditional Indian medicine as well as traditional Chinese medicine.

Medicinal plants like hawthorn and foxglove have been used to treat cardiovascular disease and hypertension. Other examples include: shikimic acid that is drawn from star anise and used in the manufacture of Tamiflu, antiviral medication that blocks the actions of influenza virus types A and B in the body; and norethindrone, derived from the wild Mexican yam, that is one of the first active ingredients in contraceptive pills. Madagascar periwinkle, hawthorn, foxglove, star anise and wild Mexican yam have contributed to medical breakthroughs including childhood cancer medicines and contraceptive pills. But all also have a proven trackrecord as food substances used in the treatment of diseases. Not only classical cultures from the past used these medications but also smaller tribal groups have developed sometimes extensive medicine systems. These systems revolve around practical applications of foodsubstances and naturally occuring tools to resolve health issues. Typical of these tribal systems is that they are animist in nature and often holist too. They are animist in that they see nature as a living entity. Living nature is filled with beings from physical substances and spirit beings of different kinds of levels of consciousness. Daoist culture roots in that same animist worldview and has trasported this to medicine as it developed. Chinese medicine in origin is an animist way of thinking. Concepts like Jing, Qi and Shen are proof of that animist nature, in that they recognize that consciousness of nature pervades all living existence.

Living existence is different from material existence persé. A car exists, but isn't alive and therefore doesnt have animation, even though it can be moved. Chinese medicine is particular as a tribal medicine in its origin, because it also used fire, stones, stickes, bones, minerals, ritual, exercise, meditation, herbs and food to affect harmony and health in natural environments. Acupuncture for instance is developed over time from massage, using bones, stones and sticks to stimulate or cut points to bruise, bleed or stimulate. We speak here of Neolithic times. In neorlithic times people did not only produce huge stone monuments and build citirs. They invented worldviews, scientific models on how the world worked, medicine systems and medical tools. Many of these are not just further developed over time, but are still in full use. When metallurgy was added to their toolbox, it made some processes more easy, faster maybe. Current Acupuncture is a very much refined technique because of the Japanese invention of filligrane needles, rooting back in the same mettalurgy already in use for thousands of years. When studying in China at the beginning of this century, we still used multiple-use needles, dealing sometimes with peaces breaking off under the skin. So convenience from the use of single-use filligrane needles now rules, but also dulling some of the massage roots of acupuncture and generating ambiguous theories on energy systems being explanation for acupuncture effects. But in Chinese medicine qi isn't energy, it is more closely related to vitality and blood.

What I like to point out here is that there is an obvious difference between natural medicine and biochemical medicine, but the difference between tribal medicine and traditional medicine systems isn't as clear for many, even though we may all understand that traditional medicine systems and tribal medicine systems all are natural medicine systems, or that tribal medicine systems likely are much older in origin than traditional medicine systems. The main difference is that tribal medicine is a specific, community-based form of traditional medicine that is deeply integrated with the cultural, social, and spiritual beliefs of a particular tribe, often involving a holistic approach to health that includes spiritual practices and community involvement. Maybe we can make a differentiation that traditional medicine systems require a literati tradition: written documents. Traditional medicine is a broader term that encompasses many systems, among which we may count tribal medicine, but also others such as Ayurveda or Traditional Chinese Medicine that use nature-based remedies and holistic principles to restore health and balance, but also have a broad sense of scientific theory and methodology. Although tribal medicine sytems do have a system of transferring knowledge from generation to generation, it is more generational dependent on how effective it is, but in a way it is also more timeless in nature, such as also nature is timeless. It is so slow in its development, that it appears frozen in time. Written knowledge allows for improvement and maintenance of improvement that tribal knowledge doesn't have.

Maybe we can pile health and medicine understandings up with tribal medicine as a root, literary history above that and methodologies on top. For instance the list I mentioned above of Chinese and Daoist medicine tools.

The best of all worlds

So healthwise, what do we need?

Our society is not structured around self management of health. As individuals we buy health related services from third parties. Healthcare has evolved from individual and tribal self-care to a massive global industry through a process of professionalization, industrialization, and technological advancement. Early self-care and traditional medicine were often based on local or cultural knowledge, but the development of modern scientific medicine as a culture of knowledge led to the professionalization of healthcare providers, the creation of formal institutions, and the industrialization of care delivery, characterized by a division of labor and standardization, and the economy of health service industries. Today, this evolution continues with digital and personalized medicine, shifting the focus toward proactive, data-driven, and individualized care. We can summarize this development as a proces of internalization to externalisation.

We have now discussed the current healthcare, traditional medicine, and tribal medicine. I have pointed out some of the negative aspects of regular healthcare, but I have tried to remain generalizing in my approach because each country has sort of its own manifested system build around the same biomedical healthcare cultural system. Many more rules and regulations than we realize are quite universal, such as your individual rights being retracted when you become a danger to your environment due to your disease, or when there is a epidemic, or pandemic, or other factors. The economic factors we discussed as being in conflict with our human rights. Pricing of means to health generates a class based society of people with or without access to health. I also pointed out that traditional medicine systems -like Chinese medicine, are not rooted in reductionist mechanics, but in common language and holist principles. With the discussion of traditional medicine and tribal medicine I pointed out the difference between histories using written sources and those rooted in the relative timelessness of tribal health cultures. It should also be noted that traditional medicine already does allow for quite a level of professionalization and caste building due to acumulation of skills and knowledge at the service of the larger community (for instance a court, village or city). Tribal health knowledge sometimes does provide the need for specialized practitioners, but like with animals, much of the knowledge and skills used to heal from disease or fracture was transferred from generation to generation within the family.

Every tribal member could play a role in the proces of self healing and group healing.

I try to be careful in saying one system is better than the other. Each approach does have clear and unclear, spoken and unspoken benefits. Science definitely has provided many new understandings, some in agreement and some deviating from past knowledge systems. It has also repressed traditional knowledge systems while heavily borrowing from that knowledge. You see that with dry needling, which in all approaches is Chinese A-Shi acupuncture, using triggerpoints for treatment. But it uses biochemical theories to explain the why and what, and -as far as I understand them, on the theory that if you hurt the system it induces self-healing, which to me is akin to the idea that torture is a healing modality. In chemical medicine science isolates substances from organics to play pool with our inner chemistry. It denies the synsergy of substances combining in an organic structure, like we ourself are the result of synergies of structiures, chemicals and substances.

Science plays petri dish with single substances while we are complex composites. Biochemical ideas are suggesting to penetrate the composition deeply and cause cumulative effects.

Traditional medicine systems have the benefit of speaking in an easy to understand language, where scientific language is often arcane and mystifying due to the knowledge barrier of higher education you have to take to understand it. Learning to apply it already takes a learning curve that can be extensive. But it's main benefit is the relationship with meanings close to life itself. Modern traditional or cultural methods often are forced to lean on scientific knowledge and culture, forcing them to betray their nature to find validation. In the Bachelor program from my school I break a lance for the idea of transculturalism. This resembles the idea that each culture is only good in understanding itself and it understands another culture only as a criticism. On the other hand we live in a pluralist world, where we can learn to become identified with another culture and thus learn to validate iton its own merits. From here we can learn that different cultures have different worldviews, and not just that, but in fact partly overlap in things they validate, and things where they disagree. For instance, modern science doesn't trust the senses, and therefore it replaces senses with instruments to observe processes and things. Chinese medicine doesn't trust instruments (historically) but it relies on emperical observation by the senses. It sees the senses as instruments, understandin g that the senses need to be trained to see things in the most pure way possible. There is a limit in what we can see with the senses, the smallest and the biggest are much closer to each other than that of instruments that can see into the macrp, meso, and the micro, or nowadays even in the nano. Chinese medicine learning specifically is based on recognizing and shaping patterns and trends in our and social developments.

Tribal medicine is different again. Developments are more random, based on trial and error, although observation definately also plays a role. We know from tribal cultures and our own pre- history that the separation between self and other/environment isn't as clear. Nowadays we consider hearing voices as pathology, but in ancient cultures it was a sign of being connected with nature. In current times that separation is also filled with the complexities of modern life, and that doesn't always provide proper incentives, and thus when hearing voices making invalid or damaging decissions is more likely. Thinking is a form of negotiation between possible pasts and futures. In a relative calm and simple reality that capacity of hearing voices can be helpful. It can create asscciation of the self with the living nature and invite that living nature in one's thought process, negotiation and decission making. Knowledge is than not owned but shared between tribal members and environment. This model is suggested in the Huangdineijing, Chinese medicine core classical text, as the manifestation of immortality.

Healthcare is, or should be a guardian of our life. One of the great modern ideas is that as a society we can all contribute to the cost and manifestation of healthcare. One of the negative development is the isolation of the user from the service through financial dependency. A combination of all these three system approaches would be great, don't you agree with me? What will it give to us?

1) the availability of complex and emperical knowledge systems,
2) the availability of mechanical tools, chemical tools and self cultivation to generate health,
3) basic generational understandings and tools that can be learned from a young age and allow for development of

preventative robuste health and stewardship over one's own health in daily life and during scrisis.

4) lower healthcare costs due to preventative self-care and thus to lower incident of disease and physical and emotional trauma,
5. a positive contribution to the level of wellbeing and social harmony in family and society.

This book, and the accompanying research are steps in that direction. We speak more of it in part 2 of this book.

PART 2

Introduction

In this part we will briefly go through the environmental risks we are currently facing. I am not assuming a doomsday protocal, but what I want to make clear that there are worst case scenario's for our future that might be here anytime. I am not going through all of them. It would take me many more pages in this book, but just a few to clarify the situation as a whole. I counterbalance that part with a brief history of this project and how it came to be, there I will offer access to questionaires to measure yourself and your health, and you can also sign up there as participant for the research. In part 3 we go a bit more into practice to help you understand the foundations of health.

I am already very happy if you bought this book as an investment in your future, You are no less than the main stakeholder in the future. In the end I do not think that rulers, govenments and companies are the only decissionmakers shaping our future. We, the anonymous autonomous individuals of the larger human and natural community also help shapiong the future. We see this in the shaping of the energy transition world wide. Even though there are political parties and economic interest groups that fight hard to stop this, it is going on under the guidance of those reeking opportunity and those with a sense of responsibility.

1: Future Risks assesment: What is the future we can expect?

As I made clear before, there are many options we face for the future. The rationale of our global village is clearly changing, and it is a matter of participation to let it move in a direction that is beneficial for all of us. I do like to press here that the future is dependent on our choices, and our choices are to be made in the present and should be rooted in what we know of the past. Internet, scien ce papers, political discussions, books and magazines, they are all ioverflowing with information and it is difficult to make the right decissions. All the scenarios I portray here are what if scenarios, based on some of the assumptions given above. I do not think I should attempt to describe what will happen if all these scenarios come true. I best let that to your own imagination. But I take it that that would be the worst of the worst scenarios.

Let us list a few scenarios:

1. *A future of rising temperatures*
   At the beginning there was the Club of Rome warning that we as people were busy altering the climate due to industrial output from our grand scale activities. It was a novelty, that was picked up mostly by a minority of the population. Industries started producing counter ideas to soften the impact of these ideas. Further research though did produce more proof of the initial manifestos. The idea was that the world would gradually warm up and that this warming would gradually alter climate zones. Several forms of pollution became visible, but cars got most of the blame in the counter propaganda. Nonetheless in 2023 there was an article in the Guardian that revealed that said that The richest 1%

of humanity is responsible for more carbon emissions than the poorest 66%, with dire consequences for vulnerable communities and global efforts to tackle the climate emergency. The most comprehensive study of global climate inequality ever undertaken shows that this elite group, made up of 77 million people including billionaires, millionaires and those paid more than US$140,000 (£112,500) a year, accounted for 16% of all CO2 emissions in 2019.

But besides this fact, our cities are on avarage warmer than their environment. Heatwaves are prolonged periods of extremely high temperatures that can lead to urban overheating and to urban heat islands (UHI). This UHI effect alters the surface of cities, making them significantly hotter than surrounding suburban and rural areas – on average 4-6 degrees hotter, and with peaks up to 10 degrees above neighbouring areas. As a result, besides becoming uncomfortable to live in, there is a pillar of heat rising from the cities, significantly altering airflows, causing climate disruptions as well.

In the last few years people speak of tipping points, after which there is no way back due to the attempt of nature to seek a balancing point. In 2025-2026 the polar ice is expected to shrink significantly and in the summer of 26 there is expected a fully icefree day at the north pole. One of the resons why they think why this is going to happen, is becasue of melting of permafrost in Canada and Siberia. As a result greenhouse gasses stuck in the ice are coming free, causing sinkholes in the landscape, but also speeding up the heating process, further melting the ice both at north and south poles, making the seawater levels rise, much landmass disappear under water. This process many researchers now see as unavoidable taking over because it produces more greenhouse gasses than we do.

2. *A future of resource conflicts*
   Resources for our survival have gotten to the point where our comfort did lead to natural degradation and exhaustion of sources. People are coming up with more and more approaches to recycling. It may be clear that nature has to be seen as a recycling biological system where due to limited space around, above and below us, there has to be a feedback system for life as a whole to sustain itself. All life and the landscape are in a symbiotic relationship. Just for that reason the ide of 'survival of the fittest' is pure nonsense. It is valid locally, but we are clearly the fittest of them all but might also be the death of it all.

   Take water. This is a water planet, but the amount of drinkable water is limited. Much water is enclosed in our cells and between our organs and in our blood. All living organisms are the same in that. The atmosphere holds huge amounts of water for moistening the world and providing drinkwater. The problem is that we use that water to cool factories, powerplants, datacenters, we add chemicals to it through our waste products. We ruin the biology of living systems and human society caused water supply scarcity is the lack of sufficient freshwater resources to meet demand, affecting billions globally due to factors like climate change, population growth, and poor management. It results in severe impacts, including poor health outcomes from lack of safe drinking water, reduced agricultural productivity, and disruptions to economic stability. Addressing scarcity requires improving water efficiency, managing sources sustainably, and ensuring equitable acces. Water scarcity causes violent conflicts. Active water scarcity conflicts include the historical and ongoing tensions between India and Pakistan over the Indus River, disputes between downstream countries like Syria and Iraq and upstream countries like Turkey and Iran over the Tigris and Euphrates rivers, and the impacts of China's dams on the Mekong River for downstream nations like Vietnam and Thailand. Local and regional conflicts are also prevalent, such as those between herding and farming communities in the Sahel region of Africa, as seen in Niger, and within the Democratic Republic of the Congo where conflict and underdevelopment impact water access.

The problem is that water isn't the only resource scarcity problem. Many of our electronics and weapens depend on minerals and rare earths that are difficult to obtain. In 2024 to 2025 we see the conflict between China and the USA growing over control over resources to keep up each's power structure and wellbeing of the population. Aging populations also cause personel shortages, which countries try to resolve through population immigration and robotification of the workforce. This in turn generates social unrest do to fear for economic refugees, forreign cultures etc. The financial resources are also limited due to the fact that a small population of mega rich controls most of the money. We speak here of 'Concentrated Ownership', with the top 1% of adults owning 43% of global financial assets, and the top 10% owning 85% of total world wealth. As a result there is also a vast inequality between the rich and the poor, where the bottom 90% of the world's population holds the remaining 15% of total wealth. This also forces us in relative poverty. Proper taxing and sharing can resolve most of the problems of resource scarcity.

3. *An AI regulated future*
   In the last few years computing power became calculation power, resulting in different forms of supercapable calculators, we loosely call Artificial Intelligence. The calculation capacity makes it possible for these systems to process gigantic amounts of data to analyse sistuations and suggest decisions. It is seductive to rely on such systems to cut corners, but in the end the reliance invites to mental stupidity of people, loosing grip on the world, and AI becoming our rulers. We cannot know yet what that future will look like. Maybe better, maybe even worse than the current world. Computers do not think like people at all. We can force them into thought simulation, but in the end they are calculators. They are not invested in biological systems. They might exterminate life as being to messy, or competetive, or it might integrate people and animals into its system, like the Borg in Startrek, or the human batteries in the Matrix. What is sure is that the qualities we have build our industry on can be better organized and used by machines then by people, so at least for a period people might become a large crown of unfed and unemloyed paupers, before a machine or population reorganizes. There acquisations that Tech Billionaires try to create an AI God, others are afraid that AI will overtake all of the economy and that large parts of humanity will be left to die off in war, hunger, unemployment, poverty, and social conflict. In the news it is sometimes suggested that these billionaires build for their own incrowd completely isolated bunker systems

for when AI takes over. Emad Mostaque from an open source AI background in a video interview[xv] suggests that about 2028/29 AI will become unstoppable if we didn't regulate its functions and existence before that time through agreements in its programming. He thinks the chance that AI will be helpful or destroy us is about 50/50 at the moment.

4. *A future in space*

   There is a lot that appears attractive about spaceflight. I am a fan of it myself. But consideringthe reality of it I am not sure what it will bring humanity. On the short terem, I do not think humanity can handle climate problems by moving to space. To actually do so there are quiote a lot of problems to overcome. The article "Medication use by U.S. crewmembers on the International Space Station" by Virginia E. Wotring in the FASEB Journal in 2015 that the environment on the International Space Station (ISS) includes a variety of potential physiological stressors, including low gravity, elevated exposure to radiation, confined living and working quarters, a heavy workload, and high public visibility. the most frequently used medications on the ISS are for sleep problems, pain, congestion, or allergy. Medication use during spaceflight missions was similar to that noted on the Space Shuttle and in adult ambulatory medicine, except that usage of sleep aids was about 10 times higher during spaceflight missions. There were also 2 apparent treatment failures in cases of skin rash, raising questions about the efficacy or suitability of the treatments used. Many spaceflight-related medication uses (at least 10%) were linked to extravehicular activities, exercise protocols, or equipment and operationally driven schedule changes. It appears that there is another problem in spaceflight, namely resource scarcity. In any size of spaceship you are required to take all your resources with you, although if the ship is big enough, with some genetic tweaking some of the resources such as food, and some organic building materials could be grown. We can conclude that under all circumstances spaceflight has to happen in an extremely poor ecological unit, and we have no idea yet how that will influence things like fertility, aging, and disease evolution. On a colony planet or moon where we have to live indoor, the first few hundred years the situation will not be better than on a ship, unless we can create huge spaces and import a huge variety of plants and animal, similar like in the story of Noah's Ark.

5. *A future in povery*

   Extreme poverty interacts with health in many ways and undermines a whole range of human capabilities, possibilities and opportunities. In 2006 Sally Murray wrote in "Poverty and health" (pubmed) that there is evidence from all parts of the world that support a link between poverty, hunger and poor child health. Poor child health and hunger in turn lead to poor school performance and therefore to a later inability to find good work and support the next family generation. Thus, Murray sees a downward spiral that maintains poverty.

   Besides poverty in itself, we can see that poverty and dependency are often intertwined. Globally, researchers have developed what is called "dependency theory" in relationships between countries. Dependency theory is the idea that resources flow from a "periphery" of poor and exploited states to a "core" of wealthy states, enriching the latter at the expense of the former. A central contention of dependency theory is that poor states are impoverished and rich ones enriched by the way poor states are integrated into the "world system". This theory was officially developed in the late 1960s following World War II, as scholars searched for the root issue in the lack of development in Latin America. This same principle is also apliccable to poor people anywhere in the world. Poor people are generally kept in dependency through dept, lack of social influence, etc. When people are suddenly becoming poor, there is little to escape that poverty, and thus it becomes circular. The cost to escape it is larger than what is available. This goes at the expense of social mobility, and increases the distance from the median between the most rich and the most poor. More poor people draws the middle class also into poverty. The reason is very easy, because dependency forces one to accept lower wages to make things end, and thus having less left to support the well being of middle class and production. Articles will become more expensive. But the main problem for a family fallen into a poverty trap, is that there is little to build a good life outside of the dependencies so that one can let go of much of these dependencies, such as costs of food, health, mental development. Refugees experience this firsst hand, but modern cities have lots of people in relative or absolute poverty. I will repeat here briefly that in 2023, the at-risk-of-poverty rate in the EU was 16.2%, which includes about 71.7 million people. While this rate has been stable between 2022 and 2023, flash estimates for 2024 income suggest a slight decrease to 16.1%. Poverty rates vary significantly by region and country, with rates above 30% in some regions and below 10% in others. These are still huge numbers, though. Poverty rates vary across North America, but a common measure is the official poverty rate in the United States, which was 11.1% in 2023, a slight decrease from the previous year. Canada reported an overall poverty rate of 12.4% in 2021, while Mexico's 2025 Gross National Income (GNI) per capita was lower than both the U.S. and Canada. In 2023, the poverty rate in Latin America was 27.3%, and the extreme poverty rate was 10.6%. We can go throughj all the continents, but what is remarkable is that besides the unacceptability of poverty, the individual in poverty gets used to it, and often takes the health disadvantages for granted. But great revolutions were always due to the extremeness of poverty. Lack of access to health and good quality of food, and lack of health education in relationship to these factors is a major issue.

6. *A future as a refugee*

From all the above it makes sense to assess your own situation and check out what is your health and wealth situation. Over time I have spoken with many people how they plan to mitigate risks. A famous one is investing in the stockmarket or crypto, both serious causes of income inequality and abuse of the economic system. Moreover, most of the things people do to mitigate povertyu isks or the risks to avoid becomeing a refugee might not be of much help if a systemwide collaps takes place. Our global culture has changed the earth into sort of an ant-nest, which has to maintain a precarious balance to maintain itself. Our whole existence revolves around survival, weather we like to recognize that or not. And survival is easyer as a group on the basis of equality and proper distribution. In equality is casued by misdirected leadership qualities on one's own behalf. Wealth then, without wishing to sound socialist, is the result of selfishness.

24 april 2025 the United Nations warned that economic insecurity, staggering levels of inequality, declining social trust and social fragmentation are destabilizing societies worldwide. The World Social Report 2025, released that day, revealed trends that are threatening communities and demand immediate, decisive policy action. The nucleus of their warning contains the following items: Over 2.8 billion people—more than a third of the global population—live on $2.15 to $6.85 a day. Even a minor setback can push people into extreme poverty, and any reprieves are often temporary. Employment precariousness is widespread, deepening economic uncertainties. Around 60 per cent of people globally are concerned about losing their jobs and being unable to find new ones. At the same time, 65 per cent of the world's population is living in countries where income inequality is growing. A large share of total income inequality can still be attributed to inequality based on characteristics such as race, caste, place of birth and family background. Without urgent action, leaving no one behind will remain a distant goal by 2030 unless progress accelerates.

Rising insecurity and inequality are undermining social cohesion and straining the foundations of solidarity and multilateralism. Over half of the global population has little or no trust in their government. Alarmingly, trust levels have been declining from one cohort to the next, indicating a systemic breakdown of social cohesion. The rapid spread of misinformation and disinformation is exacerbating these troubling trends. These factors all are like a powder keck. Add to that risks of climate disaster risks, risks on (global) war, the problem becomes visibile: all these things can make becoming a refugee the new normal.

2: Are we properly prepared?

What do we know about the world, ourselves, and the future?

I started writing this book to summarize some basic information for a general audience and to correct some missing links in current studies of East Asian exercise systems, especially the biology unserpinning things like Qigong, Taijiquan, Daoyin etc. One way or the other I never got it published. I was writing it inside a financial dry spell becasue i lost much of my work due to malversations of my clinic and school's landlord. The landlord was sort of a Donald Trump kind of power player, who thought it was more important to look innocent than to be innocent. To reorder the debts for my organisation created by this landlord's malversations I could not promote myself too much. What if the book would come out and be a success? If my healthcare project would go forward I would still not have any finances to promote it, because all would go to the debtors, of which ironically the landord himself was the meanest one.

Later the textbook content became a core e ement in the Yangsheng module of the International Oriental College Daoland Bachelor program. This module has several elements of which the book was one. The others were about how the students can put themselves into a work envornment joining esthetic medicine people. Medical organisations, alternative medicine organisations, spa's, sportsorganisations, and self organizedbusinesses. In itself this module is rather unique in Chinese medicine studies because it is normally revolving around setting up your own business as a clinic and doesn't really show the social and cultural context of the profession in east nor west.

Last year after resolving the the debt, I decided to pick up my academic career and get to do a 2nd study, a doctorate this time, making research to expand on my Bachelor study back on track to recognition as an independent university. In developing my research I found this thing in my consciousness that we are as humanity and planet in a precarious situation, where increasingly negative influences are taking over, rooted in our past and present behaviours. We discuss it hereafter before I continue with the technicallities of health.

Adressing my research purpose

By nature every human being is self-reflecting, and aiming to develop understanding of its own agency. For instance: As a Child of 9 years old, confronted with my biological fragility, born with a debilitating kidney disease, and at high physical cost barely escaped having to live connected 3x per week to an artificial kidney. As I described above, I was predicted -in spite of that escape- to not live past 40-45 years old. I was warned against doing any kind of sports to not die even sooner. When I asked about Yoga and Qigong when about 11, I got permission to do that because it wasn't taken serious as an exercise system at that time in my country, the Netherlands. Not much was known about it anyway. From Yoga I branched out to Taiji gongfu, a martial arts as well as an art of Self-cultivation and medical self-hygiene, as well as to Chinese medicine, making this field of work also part of my study at the formerly United nations allied Intercultural Open University[xvi] (now a foundation part of AZTEC Uni in Mexico City[xvii],) digging in methodologies and histories of the Chinese medicine related practices over its history. In that investigation I tried to outline the content of what makes the methods of a healthcare based upon Chinese medicine. That paper outlined different branches of activities, such as 1) qigong slow exercise and fast exercise, 2) trance based exercise, 3) qigong and daoyin/ yoga symmetrical exercise, 4) martial arts based asymetrical exercise, 5) breathwork, 6) self-massage qigong 7) comfort and therapeutic massage, 8) acupuncture, 9) ritualization, 10) worldview development. In this most of health related issues are adressed showing equivalence with modern healthcare, but then build on a few thousand years of history. The root of this is a range of developing worldview shaping theories, such as interdependency theories such as yin yang and 5 consumers (xing) theories about relatedness, where the first is a bout all things and the 2nd about living things, a proto-evolutionary theory where evolution is instant and humanity is somewhere in the focal point of that evolution by holding a middle possition, a creation theory based on the presence of heaven, earth and water realms, representing ideation, formation and life[xviii].

Now, 50 years after my operation, and about 20 years after my predicted death, I am still alive and healthy, and am acutely aware because of my results, of the fact that as a person we can do things that are not possible to be acheived by regular healthcare processes. My relative health independence was a big influence on that survival. What I learned from this is that we only need suitable tools. Suitable tools are tools in this case that are based on self-management and self- understanding. This research therefore wants to understand how people absorb exercise and experience and make the practice into useful tools. My earlyer studies helped me to develop some useful tools as teaching devises, but these tools also need further research and need comparising with existing healthcare tools to be able to scale them and convince the world of their usefulness. Key in my study is Michel Foucault's "Birth of the Clinic" description of the formation of modern healthcare from the Middle Ages to the relative present. This book really triggered me, in that it showed the attempt of medical science to take away the influence we can have over our own health. The birth of the clinic describes a certain vision of western medicinal institutes and confirms the legal authority of the medical establishement over the health and the body of the individual. I think that from the perspective of comparable histories and methods in different cultures, it is clear that this is the same in some other cultures as well, at least to a degree.

Siberian Shamans, for instance, have many different functions in Siberian societies[xix], but they are people you go to to solve some issues in health, but in contrast to that system, as a member of society you also carry your own knowledge as a family unit to solve health related issues, increasing your survival rate significantly, and limiting the range where the use of a shaman is relevant. This idea of personal (in)dependency in many cultures seem to be weighed between two extremes: self medication and medical authority. The self medication can take many forms. In most research papers self-medication is seen as taking by yourself medications sanctioned by a medical authority. But for tribal people self medication means using medical substances about which knowledge is transmitted from generation to generation. The last one, it seems, is often counted as medical illiteracy by modern science, since it didn't go through intense scientific scrutiny in laboratory testing.

C.M. Hughes et al explains: "Self-medication is becoming an increasingly important area within healthcare. It moves patients towards greater independence in making decisions about management of minor illnesses, thereby promoting empowerment. Self medication also may have advantages for healthcare systems as it facilitates better use of clinical skills, increases access to medication and may contribute to reducing prescribed drug costs associated with publicly funded health programmes. However, self medication is associated with risks such as misdiagnosis, use of excessive drug dosage, prolonged duration of use, drug interactions and polypharmacy. The latter may be particularly problematic in the elderly."[xx] The problem with this attitude is that research is primarily focussed on use of Chemical medications and regular products that might in some countries be available over the counter. It doesn't investigate other methods of self medication, nor does it take self medication out of the sphere of consumerism, which in many situations may not be an ideal solution to produce health.

The dissertation will show how in prehistoric times science, religion and healthcare were part of a unified practice of life, and that only with the advent of modern science the separation between the three became a rule. Politics governming them all[xxi]. The reason for this were adverse effects on natural health praxis judged by the now ruling medical system as perceived by psychology and medical watchers and confirmed in courts. Natural medicine systems were demoted in a reasoning where they were seen as beloning to folk religion, and superstition. All these views took an agnostic viewpoint based on the negatives but not observing the positives. Maoz dong In China experienced the negative effects of rejecting the so called 'folk-medicines', when people's health declined rapidly after eliminating Chinese medicine practitioners, and not having enough modernized medical science to replace it, since western medical science was still a relative rarety in China[xxii]. He firstly opted for a hybrid between traditional medicine and western medicine, which in Maoist terminology might be called western medicine with Chinese characteristics. This policy is still followed by Chinese medicine practice that has been developed since that time[xxiii]. Modern Traditional Chinese Medicine (TCM) is combining historically established tools within a modern scientific context, eliminating all the parts not fitting in the current scientific model, possibly being reassessed at a future date.

Doing research from 1999 to 2014 in China, I witnessed the development of modern hospitals out of the Barefoot doctors movement in China, mingling western medical science with aspects of Chinese folk and religion based medicinal practices in rural areas, and thus their development of modern healthcare-organisations, Linking with similar developments in less time in the west, organisations like the World Health Organisation etc. Like here in the west, the professional field gradually fills up every social niche. Jia Chenfu shows how the Qing dynasty (1616-1917) largely kept a hands-off policy towards public health. But for the Chinese communist state he writes: "Health and sovereignty in modern China were intertwined in such a fashion that equated a strong, autonomous nation with healthy, disciplined bodies. Individual health behaviors were linked to the status of the nation"[xxiv]. To achieve these aims, the state needed to build a health infrastructure that could manage the health of public spaces and citizens' bodies. And it needed to do so in ways that were meaningfully resonant to outside observers. Healthcare was a public status to compete with western capitalism.

European Healthcare likewise has political origins. A review of this history shows that "public health movement and a movement to reform medical science were linked to the larger social reform movement of the 1840's in Europe. It included demands for sanitary reforms, public health legislation, large scale social reforms, a reformed organization of medicine as well as a new basis for medical science. It emphasized prevention, epidemiology and social medicine rather than clinical medicine[xxv]." Nowadays it is a global industry encompassing the whole globe at the expense of native health systems on every continent, and in some cases even making them illegal to practice future proving modern healthcare[xxvi].

The dominance of modern biological, chemistry and industrial science based Healthcare science, did flourish with development of innovation, research, and offereing new services, and a high value posession of buildings and machinese to safeguard its future. The problem that I see is though that the way how modern healthcare works is mostly based on continuance of what is there, growing economic marketshare.

Risks of our modern medicine reality

This chapter reframes some of the facts we discussed before. The aforementioned are the providers of healthcare, and they stand in a triangle with insurers and patients, where the patients are both costumer and product, providing billions of revenu, holding costumers in many countries into what I interpret to be a financial stranglehold[xxvii]. The industry and insurers are both stakeholders in mainting a status quo, as well as developing a growth market. That approach also makes it vulnerable, as an industry, especially when disasters strike, and they have to rely on government funding to maintain service as good as it goes. Governments provide backup plans, ofcourse, but all of these are rooted in some form of continuation of that what is there now, which also means a quick restart from the system as it is. But what learn from modern research is that environmental disasters are slowly growing to become a bigger risk. In the European Union 87 million people run a certain risk of during their life being confronted with natural disasters like flooding, earthquake, drought, hunger, or lately a possible military- or violent social conflict.

Approximately 3.3 to 3.6 billion people already live in areas highly vulnerable to climate change, and the World Bank estimates that 1.2 billion people face life-changing risks from at least one critical climate hazard, such as heatwaves, flooding, or drought. These figures are expected to rise, as climate change is increasing the frequency and intensity of extreme weather events, leading to health crises, food and water insecurity, and displacement. The question it creates is: what if all these things happen, and then on a global scale, more or less simultaneous? Common knowledge shows that due to any form of conflict or disasters institutions run a risk to break down. Financial institutions break down, economies tumble, massive unemployement, refugees all over... In the news we often see that help only happens to arrive days after a disaster happened. Help is expensive and it often means many small donations support a part of the population. Recently in Myanmar due to civil war help was not allowed to be brought to disaster areas, In southern Turkey at the boundary with Syria there was an earthquake and disaster took a week to arrive while all structures were struck down. In japan in a combination with earthquake and Tsunamy, and a nuclear reactor out of control help was relative quick due to the relative wealth of that country, nonetheless it also relied on external help. Typhoons in the Philipines require billions to give regular relief. The wars In Gaza, Yemen, Ukrain and not too long ago in Syria, to name a few, often hinder relief to arrive, and countries sometimes even struggle to offer relief because so much is needed. If the scale of disasters and conflicts escalate, financially the burden is too large to facilitate all areas with help, or even rebuilding.

When I tell people about this they usually do not like the pessimism of this reality. But it is exactly this pessimism that urged me to write this book and do this research. The book and the research are a project of hope for a good life even after all comes falling down, if that even ever happens. It also informs the title of this book.

This book wants us to investigate if it is possible to change society and commerce enough to create an alternative health disaster and war relief program to alleviate the burden of the event on the people through preventive education and skill aquirement for situations where there is no longer anything modern available. Modern industrial medicine is expensive, and vulnerable to contamination and decay. Bonnie Dernholm points out in 2012 that: "the expiration date on the manufacturers label represents the beyond-use date for unopened products. This date does not apply after a product is opened because the broken seal and open container increase the risk of bacterial growth or cross-contamination when handled by multiple people over time[xxviii]." After a disaster of any kind risks of damage and thus contamination goes often unchecked, so as a safety precaution these medicines should no longer be used due to possible unintended effects.

This disertation as presented to the university gives the suggestion that current education for disaster relief in the population are not sufficient. Further, this research proposal makes the claim that the tools to alleviate post- or during disaster health managment are the same as reducing cost in healthcare for the population, and can be called 'socialization of healthcare through education'. The purpose of such education should relieve immedeate pressure on healthcare systems, pressure on costs for populuations and prepeare for any kind of disaster with health and survival skills anyone any place can use. The education of healthcare skills outside the norm of the industry of healthcare is in this case the aim of the study of and education of healthcare skills. The solution perceived in the dissertation based on my personal interests and vision is based on local situations, and thus individual understanding of health and the body from a naturalist perspective, using language that people can derive from experience, or that describes experience and thus allows someone to plan out a path towards health without any outside intervention or help. The methods this paper intends to investigate are methods that can immedeately be implemented and can support durable health in time of need. The primary tools to develop this, are by this dissertation suggested as an opening to better understanding to self help outside of the range of modern industrial healthcare language and instruments. The hypothesis is that people need 1) awareness of self, interior body, and their natural environment, 2) understanding of food as medicine, and 3) movement as medicine. Because these historically are key points in Chinese medicine[xxix] development.

The aim of the research is to proof the usefuness and effectiveness in health development through self-cultivation of health by supporting common people with easy methods that are without any special sport or cultural prestige, These methods should be easily learned in a period of 3 months and directly implemented in daily life. The purpose of these methods is to embed them in daily life as an ultimate form of insurance against disaster in a simular way as people have done for tens of thousands of years bu teaching adults and children to live and survive under disasterous circomstances where all support has been falling away. By doing so, the purpose is for that in daily life these skills can be generationally passed on from parent to child, and be used in bad circumstances to support recivilisation and in good circumstances it can be used for community care alike, so that communities of any kind can continuously reuse them and improve on them by learning from experience and changing environments.

The purpose of this research is to follow the learning process as well as the implementation in daily life for at least 1 year, and where possible extend the research over many years, or even a life time.

In general it has to give reasons to initiate a broad change in public mentality, and governmental guidance as to adjust society towards the possibly new realities we face.

Lars Tummers from the Erasmus university in the Netherlands suggests that government officials are sometimes experience resistence when implementing new policies. He sees five factors he calls powerlesnesses that in this paper need to be included for devising recommendations at the conclusion, based on the inferred values from the outcomes. He draws from public administration, drawing on what he calls the policy alienation concept, which consists of five dimensions: "strategic powerlessness, tactical powerlessness, operational powerlessness, societal meaninglessness and client meaninglessness". The paper considers these as factors that influence the willingness of professionals to implement policies[xxx]. So as part of the research the paper has to come up with solutions to overcome these 5 powerlesnesses.

Lets review some relevant literature

For the literature review a subselection of topics is most relevant. In the review there will be different categories of papers disscussed as leading the research. For the selected topics in the synopsis i have selected some relevant to the research.

1. *Future ecological developments as being outlined since the club of Rome sent out its warnings* and *The reality of*

economic impacts of disasters and war as seen so far and as a cumulative effect

Gifford H.Miller et all[xxxi] discuss in their Paper on Arctic amplification, the observation that surface air temperature changes in the Arctic exceed those of the Northern Hemisphere as a whole, is a pervasive feature of climate models. They point out that the albedo (reflection) of the north and south pole will diminish over time due to melting of polar ice, increasing the speed of seawater level rise and climate change over time. Preceding the melt-off of the ice, we will see that temperature warming will escape from permafrost, aggravating that trend. In the dissertation it will be tracked how the speed of climate change will affect countries according to shifting timelines and consequences.

The paper written on "Global patterns in disaster and climate risk"[xxxii], states that comparative risk information on country level is often considered of increasing importance to help steer the growing body of international finances for risk reduction, risk transfer and adaptation, especially within the emerging mechanisms for climate change-related finances. From this paper it is clear that climate change in many countries, are increasingly experiencing rise in local costs to deal with climate change, but it is also clear from papers like this that there are funds available for disaster mitigation, and these funds have the hinderance that their finances, like that of many local economies are finite.

At the "The Joint Research Centre: EU Science Hub" we are informed that in the EU about 87 million people are daily subjected to the risk of multiple environmental disasters[xxxiii], other articles give examples too about the potential risks of climate change and the economic costs it will bring to the global as well as the local society. In this paper it is not intended to discuss the truth of the matter, but the value of the possible consequences as if this were all true, and what it would mean for a future survival of humanity and the quality of that survival. The papers found on this subject in general offer a bleak image of a future that numerically seems to speed up beyond expectations with variations of the first ice-free day at the north pole within 5 year of this synopsis to 50 years, making it clear that there are now people being born that might have to live through these events.

2. *Apocalyptic stories in the media as revealing expectations*

In the last few years more and more articles appear that seem to reflect climate change. Although there are regions where people seem to be pleased with the local variation, there is also reporting on intensified severity of storms, drought etc. Unavoidable disasters like earthquackes such as a few years ago in Indonesia, Japan, Turkey, IRAN etc, are piling on top of these. The consequences of such disasters also show in political news due to reduced drinking water availability due to the overconsumption of water for growing cattle, luxury foods, reduction of rainforests around the equator changing wind river patterns, and the influence of growing citiescapes as heat pillars in the landscape also changing climate patterns. These disasters are fresh in the memory of many people. Wether they are climate changing or result of climate change isn't relevant enough, because also politically and economically there are forces at work that are in denial of the reality of all this and their consequences. Nonetheless that news cycle conflict does play out over the heads of the common person that likely is going to worry about these stories, and perhaps not know what to do about it. The growth of the threat of wars all over the globe doesn't contribute to this situation as well.

3. *Social impact of war and natural disasters on civil societies, health and disease formation*

In the context of the above the review of literature will also aim to measure the impact of war and climate change on civil society, health, and the development of new diseases. The projected global increase in the distribution and prevalence of infectious diseases with climate change suggests a pending societal crisis. The subject is increasingly attracting the attention of health professionals and climate-change scientists, particularly with respect to malaria and other vector-transmitted human diseases[xxxiv]. This and many peopers point out that change in climate will cause migration of species, but also maladjustment between species that might take generations to find natural patterns. This maladjustments is what can cause sudden change, such as an increase of malaria bearing mosquitos, change in migration patterns of locusts, or explosive growth of insect colonies with potential disastous results for our own food chain.

4. *Survivalism/elite survival vs common people survival after disasters or all out war*

The survivalist movement is a broad movement of 'preppers' who anticipate on war or disasters that are going to uproot society. Many preppers and survivalists seek for materials to use to materially survive such anticipated disasters. 3.7 million Americans classify themselves as preppers or survivalists[xxxv]. The survivalist podcast did a polling among its viewers and found that 4 topics were motivating his viewers: economic collapse, grid failure, natural disaster, and terrorist attacks. More down the line were also food shortage, civil war and worldwar, and pandamics.

Marjuna Parkkinen writes about a specific group of survivalists in Finland[xxxvi]. Parkkinen shows: 'Survivalists turn different speculated scenarios into practice by exercising the skills and knowledge they consider necessary for survival. Next to definitive grand disasters such as end-of-the-world scenarios (Rahm, 2013) and nuclear disaster (yes, even after the Cold War) (Wojcik, 1999), non- apocalyptic and temporary threats are imagined (Mills, 2019). Prepping often manifests in the collection of items that are necessary for one's defence, safety, relocation, or nutrition as well as in the improvement of social, mental and physical skills that are vital to one's survival (Rahm, 2013; Wojcik, 1999). Escaping from society and self-sufficiency are oftentimes at the core of survivalist tactics (Lamy, 1996). In this and other surveys we find that most preppers are focussing on survival with a world turning against them, and thus that there is a strong sense of self-centered self- preservation in their actions. There seems to be a lack of empathy for the less fortunate during disasters in these movements. Little attention seems to be given in most if not all of the papers to be discussed in the preview to community building or recivilizing the world, or about a world that is only half falling apart but fringing. Giving an overview of the weaknesses of current planning is a purpose of the dissertation to offer a rationale for long term planning.

5. *Literature on disaster relief and economics*

In the European Union much thought is being given to prevent pandemics as with COVID to ever happen again[xxxvii]. Rules and regulations have been set-up in the EU under the guidance of HERA[xxxviii], and likewise there are other organisations in the EU as wel as outside of the EU active in such fields.

In Canada there is recognition of the need to address growing health inequities – those disparities or inequalities in health between population groups that are systematically associated with underlying social disadvantage, is an increasingly articulated global health priority[xxxix]. These and other articles reveal that lack of social preparedness and economic preperedness for disasters is on avarage only meted out for the short term. There seems to be no long term planning in all of these researches, even though they clearly show compassion with common people. The general idea is that management of bad times will always remain a top-down engagement, meaning that the most important stakeholders, the people are left to the ability of the governments or corporations to receive what they need. To measure the limitations of what is offered is a core purpose of this dissertation to advise in the conclusions and recommendations on where the outcome of this research will contribute.

6. *Poverty and health education*

In a current article from Tulane university it is offered that: "Education gives people the tools they need to lead fulfilling lives, thrive personally, and contribute to their communities. In addition, education makes it more likely a person can access quality healthcare, find employment that pays a living wage, and live in a safe, non-polluted environment — all factors that affect well-being. In fact, people who live in lower socioeconomic conditions are at greater risk for a host of health issues, including higher rates of disease, mental illness, and premature death[xl]. The irony is that the existing broad educational programs the dissertation will discuss are all based on escaping the poverty cycle and functioning in the current economic status quo. They do not support a health independence policy of socially disadvantaged members of societies. This approach is the topic of the current research as to resolve this weakness in the current approaches.

7. *Healthcare in society, discussing past, present and future*

In the dissertation the history of healthcare has to be adressed. In a news blog from the University of York in the

United Kingdom[xli], Dr Penny Spikins, from the University of York's Department of Archaeology, said: "Neanderthals faced multiple threats to their lives, particularly from large and dangerous animals, but in popular culture Neanderthals have such a brutish and strong image that we haven't really thought too deeply about their vulnerabilities before now. "We have evidence of healthcare dating back 1.6 million years ago, but we think it probably goes further back than this." The article comes to show that Neanderthal had simple and complex care availavble, and there were signs of midwifery being part of tribal societies. From many antropological textbooks and articles it has become clear that taking care of the sick and wounded has always been part of humanity. Moreover, biologist sometimes find forms of innate understanding of herbs in animals to be used for healing or recovery. This fact is called Zoopharmacognosy[xlii]. They clarify that The concept of self-medication in non-human vertebrates wasfirst proposed by Daniel H Janzen (1978), an ecologist at theUniversity of Pennsylvania. They also suggest that self-medication by animals might be an evolutionary trait to help protect against endangering parasites. What is clear from these two references and the many other antropological source material that taking care of one's own health is a normal part of human history. What the paper wants to point out in the review that modern societies have all but erradicated value skills in self- and group-healthcare, and that self and clan or group care has always been a part of human societies and human nature. It is a normal part of human evolution and society throughout history, but current healthcare follows the thought that Michel Foucault[xliii] traced, namely that modern healthcare science and institutes see themselves as the authority over the human body, while common people are seen as incapable to understand biology. This research project is going to try to proof that it is possible to build relative modern tools that do not require specialized biological, chemical or technological knowledge to take care of general health while reducing health dependency on third parties such as medical doctors and hospitals, following the argument that people managed to survive for millions of years. What the program tries to do is restart that history and improve on it in a systematical and scientific fashion. For this I will make use of the Kuhn cycle. The Kuhn Cycle is a simple cycle of progress described by Thomas Kuhn in 1962 in his seminal work "The Structure of Scientific Revolutions"[xliv]. Kuhn challenged the conception of science, which was that it was a steady progression of the accumulation of new ideas. He saw science more like a spiral or cycling development where renewal takes place, meaning that science also has to continuously cycle back to its roots to review itself. In the preview we will discuss the role of what Kuhn calls Pre-Science and contrast this with the ideas on science that he discusses. It also tries to contrast the benefits and weaknesses of present and premodern healthcare systems.

8. *Review of healthcare effectiveness as preview control group as norm vs research outcomes*

Part of the preparation is based on review of articles offering data on healthcare effectiveness. This is data driven research on issues such as the application of insurance companies or the absence of insurance companies, the impact of 'pay out of pocket services', and what people trend to do in anticipation of health related issues and how useful these are. These papers which are very fragmentary and disease-topic sperated researches often seem to focus on cost-effectiveness over actual success rations of Healthcare, and The paper has to research an explantation for the effectivness of general healthcare in figures[xlv]. [xlvi]

9. *Literature on healthcare history and methods*

There has to be a section investigating the observation of healthcare in animals, healthcare deduced from archeology, tribal medicine, prehistoric medicine, history of Chinese medicine and its paradigm shifts over time etc. These papers will be analyzed using the Kuhns cycle of paradigm shifts in medicine and science[xlvii]. In this the paper looks for an argument to state that the current capitalisation of health is but an abberation of historical use of healthcare, and the Kuhn Cycle of scientific development aims to be applied in resoning that adaptation of the current system into a non capitalized system is a form of progress and necessity.

10. *Biological evolution driven by behavior and environment,*

Chinese medicine plays a role in the biology or nurture discussion, because from over 2000 years ago it reasoned that self-cultivation by means of particular methods have an effect on the civil and biological success of individuals to live longer[xlviii] where the argument for this program leans on the dominance of nurture using biology through training of the body and the mind, using articles focussing on discovery in epigenetic adaptation of evolutionary traits in animals[xlix], s.a. on the results of epigenetic change in mice, but also how poverty, environment and wealth affect health[l] on how socio-economic circumstances generate differences in biology and social endurance. This part of the review will provide some of the rationale for the current research on which the hypothesis of its effectiveness is based.

11. *Existing experiments in healthcare related to my research*

The thesis review will also discuss research done in alternative and complementary medicine and what are some of the strong points in this research, and how these outcomes may apply to the use of this research program to benefit future users. This part will also be included in the material for the participants to help them understand what they do and how it will benefit them.

The research gap

A research gap is what in science is called an area that has not been extensively investigated. It is certain that a lot is spent on maintaining the status quo after disaster. The focus is on the continuation of nation states and economic power to manage affairs. But there is no substantial focus on the needs of the individual. This book and the research is focussed on the singleminded needs of the individual and family or community unit independent of money, government protection and so on.

State promotion of civil protection is rooted in stacking emergency packages. Besides these emergency supplies not being endless in volume for most people, disasters usually have long tails. Insecurities about housing, health and food are going to be major concerns. Personally I hope things get that far.

There is a big movement called "Survivalism", we get to talk about this elsewhere, but suffice to say that survivalism as it is just isn't available or suitable for everything. The main takaway from this is to learn wild camping, and to live from the land.

The third aspect governments and society adviocate is taking Insurances, which means spending funds on something that might not be able to pay out something valuable to you at the time of occurence. He survivalist takaway probably is the best of the three, because it allows you to immedeately develop a mobile lifestyle as a refugee. But this program wants to leverage particular required knowledge about health in that situation, when your meds and bandages are long gone already.

The topic contains many aspects related to self care in crisis situations, such as after natural disaster, war, extreme poverty etc. Self regulated healthcare or management of health with shared skills between family members or social group can provide securities in times of need when regular healthcare is unafordable or not available. This first half of the 21st century gives ample opportunity for a global crisis of unknown proportions, and study of methods in healthcare that can support human wellbeing in such circomstances is of prime importance.

In existing studies the emphasis is on the continuation of the availability of regular healthcare and medicine under all circomstances. At the same time the threats of climate change, economic collaps and war when viewed in light of experience in the last 50 years shows the risk of longer time unavailbility of support for parts of the world after such issues and that rebuild if it happens can take many years where health and civilization can easily degrade into disease, abuse, and violence. Here we also find the Study Gap. There is hardly any research to methods in existence that can be used to prepare people for global risks that will help people be healthcare independent in a way that people have done forever before the present market regulated period of healthcare. As such, the review of literature suggest that this might be a Blue Ocean research, and such be groundbreaking, while serving as an example for development of comparable research, and the development of practical educational products.

Mehodological research of methods, reception and retainment of methods is the prime goal of this research that focussing on 3 approaches from Chinese medicine history that are low tech, easy to learn and apply, and this at almost no cost for the user under the right conditions. From here it can inferred how these methods when succesfully deployed can contribute to people's wellbeing in times of need. The findings will not offer solutions for specific diseases, accidents and so on. The outcomes will focus on general succes of a disciplinary application of exercise, ways of gathering and eating foods, and awareness training.

What i think is of great value in this program is the occurence of the following as motivational factors. In brief:

1. increased fear in society for the future (realism vs irrationality, fear for climate change, fear for war, fear for natural disasters, fear for economic ruin, fear for ill health/burnout/autoimuune diseases)
2. need to be prepared (rationality of social preparedness)
3. need for more affordability in healthcare and something owned by population and not subject to commerce

This book already offers some solutions, but the accompanying research takes it further. The objectives/research questions within the context of the before are:

1. Is and how is the daoland healthcare program a good addition or alternative for regular healthcare?
2. What factors will add to the effectiveness of the program and make it suitable as a foundational healthcare for family use and generational transmission?
3. Does the program reduce healthcare dependecy and reduce cost in healthcare, especially in times of crisis?
4. Will the program have good family retainment through the generations when presented as such, especially in crisis?
5. Are people willing to change health habits when alternatives are concretized that can be transfered

from generation to generations, and create a general prepearedness for great life changes in society for lower costs than regular healthcare?

I already assume -ofcourse- that it is going to work because I have seen it work for many people in different kind of circumstances. But now we plan to put clear numbers and value on it, so that we can help everyone battle the negative spirals of global society and learn to be prepared in worst case scenarios, and to generate policy advises for social change.

The hypotheses of this work are:

1. Society isn't properly prepared for eventual worst case scenarios in regard to war and environmental degradation
2. (relative) Poverty in many countries causes reduced access to healthcare, therefore it is of the greatest importance to develop a healthcare that is accessible to everyone for little or no payment, and the way to do that is through revision of cultural medicines
3. Foundational healthcare should be simple, not require scientific learning and be transfereable from generation to generation

PART 3

The Daoland research project

To test your health

In Chinese and western perspectives on health and what a people should be able to do to call itself healthy there are some differences. Yanghseng is the Chinese way of seeing health as a program of achieved health in spite of possible disease or handicap, while in western vision you have either health or you have a handicap or disease, but you might be in relative well-being. These two visions differ significantly in onset and implications. That is what this book is about. It is about introducing alternative perspectives on developing healthy on the basis of what we might call 'culture diving'. It is an investigation in practices and belief systems. Fact is that all our beliefs in what we know are programmed by the culture we live in. we go look in another perspective and see if that perspective can work for us or how we can make it work within our own belief system. This cultural diving we call becoming member of Daoland. It implies that we learn to make choices about what we belief and can do. It is the natural consequence of living in a global society that beliefs in results.

Part of any yangsheng healthcare program is not to battle your symptoms but to help restore the ideal of vitality and life so that your natural health can come about and symptoms can fall back into the fold of health by themselves. Yangsheng is not therapy, it also is not anti-therapy. Yangsheng is about taking life as a garden or a little child and tending it until it grows strong and fruitful. So what is it that is ideal?

Look at the following list of achievable life and health qualities to have an impression of things you can test yourself on in relationship to what yangsheng healthcare considers a healthy situation. Health is what is continous in us. Disease is what degenerates us. Health has little to do with our ideas and opinions. Science also has a difficulty being clear about health. Science is just a rating system giving an estimate of the result based on your survival chances in common circumstances. It creates a story to live by. And so does Chinese medicine. Science is a story to pep you up or to depress you depending on the judgement. In The Daoland Yangsheng vision your current health is a starting point, and from there we gradually cultivate step by step to bring you up. For some that will be faster then for others, but some slower people become bigger masters in living and surviving, in florishing even, than others. Ideally you see it as not belonging to a particular school of thought, but a tool where the tests objectifies the range of your body's well being. We want to measure our changes in capacities, and use that to improve on ourselves.

These are links to questionaires about your health. Participation is free (no charge!) and voluntary, although I think that if you already bought the book, you can as well test yourself. It also gives you opportuntiy to link in as stakeholdere in the research. They will give you a score on which you can found a good assessment of your health and what qualities you need to improve your health.

These qualities are ofcourse based on activities within the Daoland Healthcare program, but, we will also focus on the research program. Besides that, on the basis of the descriptions of the Daoland Yangsheng program in part 1 it should be easy to see what is available to you in your own surroundings in case you do not like to commit to this not for profit program.

Mobility health: https://forms.gle/XQqk8auRZZEkgUSZ8. In the paper version of this book, please fill in then adress in your search machine. In this form you are asked to do some basic practices to test your range. You will receive a reply with suggestions on what to pay attention to. You will also receive an advice what practice in the Daoland program is available for you to practice at the moment. In the research these practices in general refer to the kind of mobility we develop in Wudang Agility fitness

Male health: https://forms.gle/ofyTuQkuLGKudBMm7
Female health: https://forms.gle/7gK1YxDW9D4r89uy9
General Health analysis: https://forms.gle/jXGrB6tCrtHYgvJe8

All the forms are going to be anonimized for research purpose. You will in the research get a number assigned for your interviews etc. For reference you get a copy of your answers sent back and later when you enter the research we will finetune your program using the outcomes you recieved to keep it separated from the research data.

My suggestion would be to do every day one test, you whole family can do it, and in 3 days you are ready. You can also do them in one sitting. It doesn't matter. Important is that you are truthful in answering. Your outcome will replied automatically. The data we use for our research and is only anonymously used. Your name and the date are going to be immedeately separated by a randomizing program. You will get a number that you can fill in in any other time you fill in the form. Our research will take some time to complete, but if you can fill it in after a half year and after one more half year it will provide us with all the date we need: with 'we' I mean you and me. You can compare the outcomes and see what improvements you made.

In the next chapters we are going to work on the development of a general understanding of health, and how to carry yourself for that purpose.

The points in the tests give you a general quality marking indicator to measure if you are on average fit or not. Ofcourse you need to do two things before you fill it in. Sign in so that your data can be sent to you and you need to use the key given at the end of this book to show you how to rate yourself.

There is more than being fit as to be able to move easily. In general one naturally feels hopeful and curious about life, is every day active, doesn't eat too much or sleep too much as there are other factors that prove one's fitness. But how to determine one's fitness and what one can work at?

Firstly: with every question you have to ask yourself what should be possible and in how far you are able to fit in the answer of the category. The yes and no answer is very black and white on purpose.

Secondly: you have to count the difference between yesses and nos. if the difference is high in favor of the yesses, you seem to do good. If the odds are stacked to the no's favor you seem to do not so good. In the case you now start worry, all these things are addressed deeper into the book with suggestions for what you can do. It will explain aspects of fitness and how to get there.

Important to the program is the understanding that nobody is hopeless in achieving health but that change usually is gradual due to the natural ability of the body to adapt its form to habits. Habits create patterns of formation to the body both in a good and a negative way. The way of health therefore is about monitoring habits, generating good habits and understanding what is actually good or bad in this context. The obvious is not always the correct. People usually live by myths on things. One thing to remember is that developing health also means developing an understanding about health. Health never comes about without a certain amount of study and practice. First now we need to study the importance of culture. Culture is the single most important factor in developing understanding.

The differences between eastern and western approaches to health are obvious. For one, the Chinese approach asks you continuously to test yourself against what should be possible for people, while the western ideas of health is continuously measured to possible deviations and handicaps that have happened to you. The eastern approach emphasizes what should be, while the western approach emphasizes what is there now. The eastern approach is goal oriented and does not accept disease or handicap as a given, while the western approach is generally accepting and remains centered on the permanence of handicaps or disease. Another difference is that in western health culture our personality is seen as a permanent presence, never minding our problems and how much they hinder us. In Chinese health culture problems are seen as altering our personality and the sense of responsibility we should take as a basis for our actions. Disease then is taken into the same category as drugs and helping us to falsify our perspective on reality. Another way of putting is that our problems take over our personality and demonize us by forcing us in to selfish (wanting, angry or fearful) behavior, which in turn undermines our health. Modern neurological investigation seems to confirms this vision. The vision suggests that we are the result of what we ingest, allow ourselves to feel and think, how we behave and talk. From biological perspective we are willing to fill in the blanks on what we did not perceive and make p ideas about ourselves or what we perceive or know that are not necessarily true or helpful.

Although this seems a gloomy perspective on being human to some, in fact it is our reason to be hopeful about our future.

It means that problems we face are things we can deal with, and when not capable of solving them, at least managing them to a degree that they contribute to our health and pleasure in life instead of being a constant source of annoyance. Practices such as taijiquan, yoga, qigong and so on exists by the grace of the nature of being human is like this. They help develop health almost accidentally due to the process of continuous self-practice and self- investigation. Self- practice and investigation is a process of self-generation. We can call the learning process one of 'accidental intentionality'. Focus on health development is not going to do it for you. Healthcare in any form isn't a science, it is an action. The process starts -though- with asking oneself questions and be fair in answering them and not pass their consequences too lightly.

These seem simple enough explanations but it is by no means enough to really explain the why's and how's of health. It shows that health is:

- *Partly a capacity that requires practice to develop and maintain and that if nothing is done gradually withers away and degenerates*
- *Partly dependent on cultural views and how they make us relate to ourselves and the world around us, so that people need cultural training to be healthy*
- *Relates to us as a developing person and therefore relates to our morality and how we feel successful in life*

Believe it or not, although these issues seem obvious ones, in this modern world discussing them or taking things like health in personal control are for most people taboo issues. They seem to contradict our mechanized worldview that by taking chemical or herbal medicine or having surgery done (all by means of third party judgment and intervention) you can also undo disease. Especially the last issue can cause people to feel conflicted. In most cases after regular treatment of disease scars, handicaps and loss are being faced. Regular medicine in that sense is battlefield medicine. It has to help us going, but not necessarily for our own benefit so. Looked at our health from this perspective shows the unreasonableness of our behavior and the undeniable failure of the modern healthcare system, even if it lets drop mortality rates. We have to ask us if the price of added discomfort is actually helping.

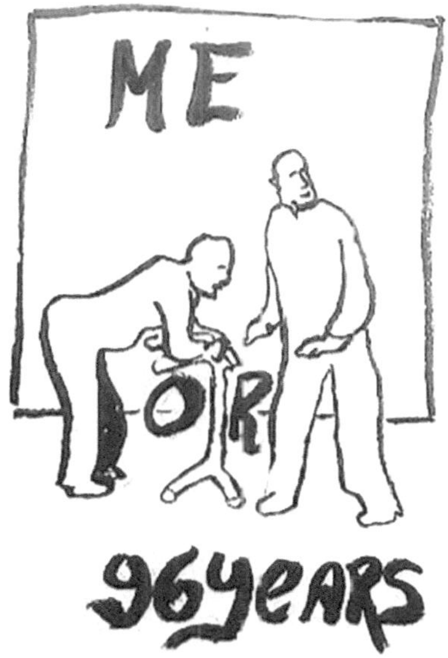

The program should be extended with health study for lay people. To help change ruling attitudes about this was one of the reasons why people asked me to publish. So to write a book in a simple and concise way about this issue is not an easy task. In fact I have to explain things from the ground up, much in the way how popular publications are driven by simplicity and intuitive accessibility. But in opposition to simple and intuitive statusquao confirming explanations, we have to get out of that box, and learn to allow incremental random changes to manifest themselves to build understanding. Developing health isn't a lineair proces.

Health is not a popular matter though. Health is often an excuse to have a nice time, being together with others, a bandage for loneliness. Health practices effectiveness is hard to prove by means of statistics as long as health practice is not a common daily practice. The results can only be tested on hindsight, and the results of the one do not need to be repeateable by another. The occurrence of accidental success does not generate convincing science because it does not count in the people who are not motivated by themselves or their environment to set it through and reap the actual benefits of taking care of themselves.

Taking care of one's health requires one to develop an attentive and somewhat analytic and intuitive mind. Researching and developing one's health is not a fashion fad that comes and goes with the seasons. Health is a prerequisite to live well. Ofcourse we can have satisfying lives too when handicapped by debilitating disease. People can be magnificent tin how they cling to their lives and are able to maintain a helpful temper. But this life situation means we have to commit to a lot of work if we also wish to be independent. That work goes at the expense of what we otherwise might have achieved. As a person we therefore by nature require to put effort in self-maintenance, much like how cats and dogs groom and stretch themselves in a sort of nature given yoga and qigong play.

There are the seasonal changes that drive us to alter ourselves and adapt. Therefore, while writing the book I took several things in consideration:

- *What is useful for people to know about healthcare, such as that you yourself are the most suitable person to take care of yourself and that you should have practical tools on how to take care of yourself.*
- *Then also what is weak in the current popularization of yangsheng healthcare, such as the lack of information organization or organization of healthcare workers under one unified idea due to the entrepreneurial involvement of practitioners*

- *Why are there so many fraudulent or ignorant people carving out such brilliant careers in this profession. Moral professionals by nature unify and co-operate, have no ideas that separate them from history and unifying theories, do not charge more than that could include the not so affluent to participate*
- *Other factors,*

For this reason the book does not come alone. It comes with training programs, informational courses on introductory, a semi-professional and professional level (do not forget that to be healthy is a profession!), a website where one can share ideas, networks in social media to help develop mutual sharing and development that allows the individual to build a sound healthcare system around and within them, generate insurances for support and where possible even developments for localized financial insurance (currently under investigation and experimentation) for natural healthcare. Healthcare is not only the activities you can do, but also the professional site of it, the support network, feedback programs and so on. The most important things is that all these things contribute to health. Taking healthcare in your own hand then also contributes to your sense of accomplishment by the awareness that you help generate healthy natured jobs, even of it is because you eventually choose to work in healthcare and education yourself.

Chinese Medicine Healthcare is experience based. That means that every person manages his or her own experiences, that does not mean that anyone is experienced and therefore have authority. Even the most experienced eventually dies and that means experience is not sufficient. Health is a practice of daily trial and error while maintaining long time overviews.

It is of importance to realize that:

Healthcare refers to health and not to solving problems and treating diseases.

Disease-care as functional in modern hospitals is created for that purpose. Watch my language here. Based on other cultures I change the meaning from activities in hospitals and by physicians to 'disease care' while I point out that what we people who are specialized in supporting health promoting activities belong to healthcare.

The thing is that explaining practices in itself doesn't mean much. Practices have to come together with ideas. Most ideas are fixed within a system. Because of the cultural aspect of health, healthiness does not exist in the isolation of one person. Health is a shared commodity. Health is partly based in understanding what we would be if healthy.

A summary of things you can do to increase health does not give you a handle on how to develop health. Skills by themselves do not produce health. Skills need context. Context consists of theoretical ideas, a goal and personality development.

When doing things for health that keep you busy but passively so, you probably increase your health a bit, but it is an inefficient way of dealing with health. Developing health is more of a science than is treatment of disease. Disease is helped by trial and error. You win some and you lose some, because all diseases are a bit unique. But health is the same for all people within one cultural model and biologically so somewhat similar too, because whatever biological model we follow in any culture: every time we find out that in health we share the most similarities. But considering our motivational part we require culture to reach for the goal of health. So becoming more healthy requires us to become more culturally developed. This coursebook leans towards application of Chinese cultural views on health that can be easily combined with the views of your own culture. The skills are in origin quite Chinese, but their application certainly belongs to the modern world.

My complaint about 'passive participation in activities' can be seen around us. Also it is easy to see how it does inefficiently contribute to health you see this in sport centers where people slave themselves on machines. Although for a while they radiate vitality, they are also prone to burnout, heart attacks and depression. So their sport program did not generate fitness, it generated battlefield fitness, where bodies are seen as expendable.

Also we see that there are scores of people who practice things all their life and still obviously look unhealthy and often are so.

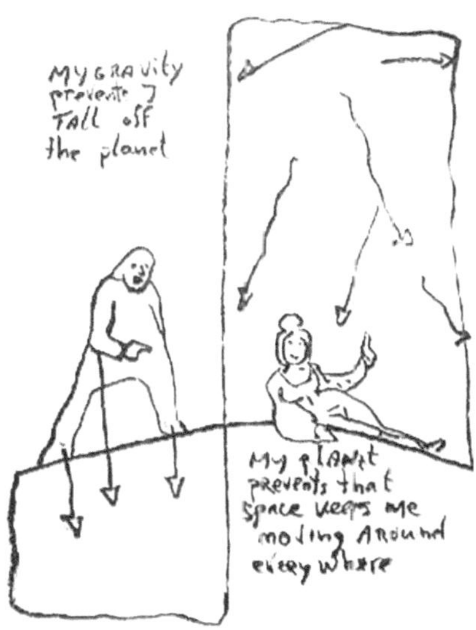
My gravity
prevents
fall off
the planet
My planet
prevents that
space keeps me
moving around
everywhere

Health-practice is based on the understanding of principles, so it is impossible to develop one's health without study. Some principles we act from naturally so due to our being member of a culture. But the understanding of this culture often is only sketchy, and so is therefore our health. Healthcare is not just following principles. Principles belong to a culture with defined visions on what is health and how practices fit in that culture to achieve those ends. When seen from another culture these practices might even look naïve, too elaborate, complex or even superstitious. Seen from Chinese medicine biology sports-center-fitness and even many team or partner-sports that have developed in the west the last 150 years or so are typically unsuitable to generate health.

I have to warn you. It is not in the nature of cultures to be tolerant about ideas prevalent in other cultures. It is also why in western societies Chinese medicine and other naturopath medicines are tolerated but not accepted. The tolerance is based on pluralist principles, which means that they are only allowed to be understood by means of a dominating culture. Appreciation of other cultures is based on principles of equality. Understanding takes place inside civilized people. There are usually only a few civilized people around, and the statement of this book is that civilized people are also healthy people. They can live without regrets because they treat everyone and everything as equal to themselves. To be civil is a conscious effort you have to undertake every day. Most people are civil at times, but rarely all the time, because we are also ruled by our confusions. Our confusions can look quite straight forwards. You may be surprised how much of our certainties are in fact constructed without a ground of reason or realism. It is a human thing. We feel safe in certainties, even if they are just assumed certainties. Culture helps us to stay within a fold of certainties, so that even if we go all astray on things we can find our way back to health.

People normally do not have a choice to which culture they belong. It implies that they do not have too much free choice to believe whatever they want too. But in this time of global migrations we get to taste in many alternative ideas. Many of those ideas are much more wise than the ones our own culture produced. Other cultural groups think the same about our culture. Every culture has things to offer. In equality that can be celebrated.

In mirroring cultures we learn to understand more about ourselves and the culture we belong to. Being cultural, or being part of a culture requires one to make conscious effort and choices. It also allows us to switch cultures, as long as we manage to develop a consistent switch. So the Daoland program is not to make you believe in Chinese practices over non-Chinese practices, it is about developing cultural awareness as a prime directive in developing health. It is about understanding how awareness of proceedings of the body helps to give directions to the workings of our body so that we may manage them properly instead of leaving them to decay over time due to negligence. So, in writing this book on health I knew I have to point out the influence of culture and cultural views to make ideas and practices from an alien culture as the Chinese acceptable to westerners, or maybe Africans and natives in the amazon rainforests too. To be all folklorizing by giving you sketches of wuxing and yinyang mechanisms as other books usually do would not really contribute. These books have their use, but in effect they do not show you what is Chinese about it, they just show you they have strange ideas that sound exotic but which we cannot really comprehend because they seem to relate to things we know and they seem not to. It is in this borderland of knowing and not knowing where we come to study cultural difference and thus learn to appreciate ideas about health and what they actually imply.

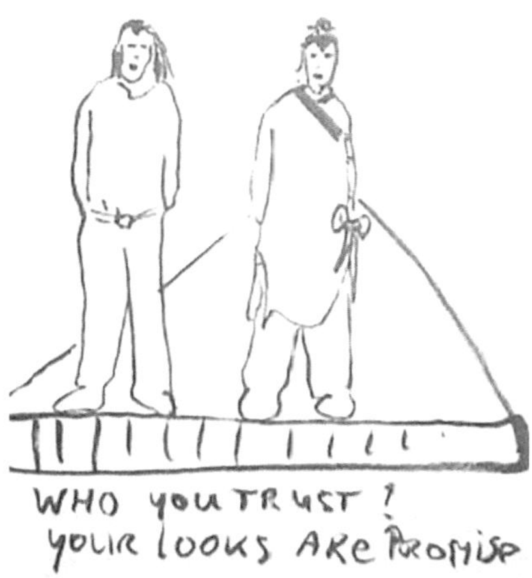

I have been living and studying the last decennia between cultures. The Netherlands is almost all my life a multi- cultural melting pot. Recently our right wing government has decided that the Netherlands should be a monocultural meltingpot where only Dutch-ness can prevail. The Netherlands is also experiencing lots of people burning out under stress, increasing discrimination levels and racist and religious violence. You may ask yourself questions if the belief system creates the problems... Culturally it is a mess. Like in England and other countries we see a whole new culture coming into being as a result of mixed ideas which on both sides are not fully understood.

In the USA we see the nation is gradually shifting from an anglo western culture model to a latin western culture model, while in Arabic countries culture shifts from a western despotic model towards a sharia based western democratic model. In China we see that the eastern imperial model has shifted via an enlightened despotic cultural model to a pluralist Confucian civil model. I have made frequent visits to some America's both on the Anglo and the Spanish sides, and since over ten years I lived in more in China among Chinese people and not westerners than among my students and clients that I used as experimentation control groups. In the recent ten years people on both sides started questioning where I belong. Since I normally dress up in my monk's attire I am very well aware of the aspect of representation in people's mind eye. The suit works very much as an exclamation mark that makes some anxious about me and others feel in trusted hands. It is a sign that visual cultural differences triggers inside people's awareness that are significant and require deep investigation. Our looks are just as much part of language as are our words and behaviors/postures.

We also see this happening in the world at large, in political and international conflicts. These are all based on cultural differences that lead to misunderstanding and misrepresentation even while everyone has the best intentions in mind (according to their own cultural mindset). Health works exactly that way. You have to study culture to be able to develop health. Disease might be personal, but health is a cultural thing, like science, art and religion.

In the process of living between cultures I have observed how I changed and how my judgment on things changed due to assimilation of alien cultural ideas and habits. I also observed people in how they deal with information and experiences in different cultures. I have also witnessed the enormous strides scientific knowledge has made, but that while science is not dealing with a multicultural world other then as an observer with a relative blind spot for its own cultural roots and branches. On this all I can only say that culture matters. In any country, culture, rules to live together they should be clarified in every level of education and should be a major part of education to help create harmonious societies, because study of culture lines out what does it mean to be civilized, being human, being happy and being healthy. And as such I came to realize that being civilized and being healthy go together very strongly. For people learning to be civilized includes people to learn be healthy and have strong principles of personal hygiene. Also a disadvantage of modern society is that being civilized is not part of the common c.v. of our educational program, so too often we are cultured or mannered but not necessarily civilized. Lots of our actions we consider 'culture' are in fact folklore and mannerist, if not, then not well understood.

Concluding: I think health study and being civilized are an integral part of what a culture offers. That was so for the ancient Greeks and Romans, but also for the Chinese and Koreans. It also rings true for us modern westerners. Lack of modern time is that we are not so systematic about it, so we do not really study our culture as a fixed part of our lives and we are not guided to be part of our culture or any other culture although we do flirt a lot with things cultural or health. We often wait until society becomes fully distorted before we start protesting negative change. We ask the army to intervene or politicians or the police. We did not live together in a mature enough way that most problems could be prevented. The same we do with our health. We know we are aging so we can predict things to happen to us. We do not prepare for it other than taking an insurance, which is a bit like betting on a horse: you cannot really win because you know that everybody trying to help you also is trying to make a living build on helping you and you are the one paying for that help. Medicine is in that sense a lot like mustard that is offered after a meal has been eaten. I do not mean to say that medicine isn't useful, but medicine is a last resort issue. Prevention is the real medicine, and prevention is in education, practicing oneself, learning, dealing with things and so on.

The thing is in healthcare there is one main interested party only, that is we ourselves and thus healthcare is or should be a shared interest between all people. Although some commerce is naturally involved, the primary goals should be humanities ability to survive and flourish as a species and a part of greater nature. Our personal goal to live happy and satisfying lives is identical to the goal of all humanity. It also means that by making sure we ourselves are healthy we are involved in working at the wellbeing of all people, other beings, the environment etc.

In fact the also foregoing is part of the United Nations charters on healthcare that drive the development of the Daoland Healthcare program we will discuss in this book.

Daoland is called Daoland because it wants to describe the experience of health and what you can do yourself to develop health forward. Health is not something people have, they create. The Daoland courses, trainings etc are to help ourselves and each other to validate health and promote skill development in preventing problems to get out of hand. For instance why go to a myofascial masseur if smart dynamic stretching does the job better? Why take a painkiller if mobilization of our joints and muscles in gentle exercise improves circulation and relieves the pain more effectively? Why go for a liposuction or knee surgery when overweight if you also can move and learn to re-appreciate your methods of eating, breathing etc to enhance fat-burn and restoring healthy body form.

As modern people we are all children of history as it plays out in modern times. History is not only facts, but also politics, language change, fashion, feelings and so many other factors. We as individuals help shape that history by what we do every day. Our actions allow heroes to do their things while making the world better, but our things also allow villains to do their things and make our world an unhealthy place to be. Nothing bad can happen to the world if we all take positive action in our private spheres. We do not need to wait for others to do so. If we look for environmentally or socially helpful careers, for watching programs that inform us well next to the ones we watch for scare and other thrills, for rectifying ourselves when we find our judgment or action is in error...

Modern people with all the good that is within us, we are also thought to be big children and thus too often childish, dependent and ignorant. The availability of knowledge so far has not brought us maturity but it does nourish our stubbornness. Although it allows for more people to be involved in our human development it also makes every voice individually more easily lost in the mass of voices. Attractiveness then is a major element in making yourself heard. Attractiveness is often based on good looks and recognition of what we intuitively feel to be right. As publishers put it: if it isn't fashionable it will not sell. These things are addressed in this book.

Unfortunately healthcare is not by itself fashionable. What is fashionable are tips and tricks. Publishers seem to think that people interested in health are stupid and not interested in understanding things. That is at least what several publishers made me clear in the past.

Fashionable information is based on maintained confusion and dependency. If confused everything sounds acceptable as an exit from confusion. Here we also reach a critical issue in Chinese healthcare thinking, namely that the dedication and moral stance towards care from distributer and student is essential in the process of developing health. To achieve health you need to want health and be willing to dedicate yourself to the process.

Health is often mystified by healthcare implying or suggesting self-help books and people who sell products to make you healthy. But in fact you yourself are a closed book when you follow such books. For this book this also creates some sort of paradox. The point of this text is to help you open yourself as if you were a book, and outline some basic principles you can follow in your pursuit of health. Ofcourse, the Daoland program is initiated to share knowledge and skills between people and people buy into the program to help the sharing process. When people come to take a Daoland massage, facelift or follow a fitness program or something they also buy something. But like with western medicine we try to build a diffuse cloud of skills and knowledge that does not require a bright example/ guru or something at the top. Daoland is meant as a path of self-discovery where some boundaries are set to help you discover how much you can or ought to do. This way the

Daoland healthcare system does serve to generate a tool that is equally accessible to everyone to develop and obtain health.

This text then, although it shows some exercises too is not a practice book or advertisement in the common sense. It is a help book to make everyone a health scientist of sorts. It also helps to see healthcare in the context of open source programming, gaming etc, things that many people are involved in for fun, but that also help develop skills useful in healthcare, if only people would see themselves as bodies and in the context of the world as a whole.

So this book is in fact a book to help you develop fun in life, but then a fun based on ability and knowledge about yourself and fellow beings. Please, enjoy it. Become a Daoland Citizen..

The computer game metaphor in health

When experiencing ourselves we see that there are many factors present. In fact these factors form story lines. Story lines can be influenced, but we need the right metaphor to influence the outcome.

Interviewing people who take psychotropic drugs the attraction is that the narrowing of their consciousness makes them experience the wholeness of their life within a certain context. Much of the Americas traditional spirituality is focused around that experience. In fact Tibetan Buddhism and even Daoism consider life stages much as secluded unities with begin, middle and end. It makes that life is experienced as both space and time defined by events unfolding or caving in on themselves, summarized by the magical word 'change'. The awareness of the limitedness of life as a space is a very important one because it allows us to time alterations we see happen in the whole of our life. Ofcourse we do not know if we are going to live long or short lives, if we go have many diseases and pains or not. We just hope for the best. But watching ourselves in the envisioning of the whole of our life makes the experience or presence of health and life very immediate and a pressing matter. That makes the influence we can have on the personal healthcare a process much like gaming. And because it feels like that we feel like cheating in one way or the other hoping that we can alter the stakes in our favor. If the health deteriorates we feel cheated by the game. In fact we see more people being cheated by the game then people who win. Why is that? It is because people cheat by giving the game out of their hands, they gamble by means of hoping that their insurance will cover the costs of 'fixing' them. But that is not cheating, that is passive suffering. I am not saying people should skip their insurance or national healthcare plan; they are after all intended to be a safety net. Cheating is taking things in your own hand and leveling the playing field, so that you improve your chances on having a long and good life. If habits do not help to get a good life, you generate new habits that do. It also means that you can rely on self-generated second chances to develop improvements on yourself. The body changes slowly and learns equally slowly, so results showing error or success sometime s take time to mature. Learning to recognize that process helps one to understand the process of health changes early on and alter your strategies. You will find after some time you need few tools only, don't need special medication or specialized help in more than half of what can happen to you. That safes you on your medical and insurance bills, so these are like bonus points. Live life like you are a SIM I would say.

In Chinese medicine the experience of health and self is often translated in the metaphor of a country. Therefore we also use the metaphor of a country for how we relate to each other.

Anyone active in the Daoland Healthcare reality SIM therefore is designated a Daoland citizen. In time when we become large enough we could organize ourselves like a real country, developing passports, coinage, mutual support programs and so on. We can help our national governments develop true healthcare policies as well as understanding between peoples from different origins. I think No country should be ruled anyway on other premises then achieving happiness, healthcare and future prospects on improvements. Savings, possession and so on is all nice, but too often they cause disease, stress and other things weighing us down. Societies as they now exist ofcourse are old fashioned, conservative and do not have individual needs at the core of their minds.

Understanding of human potential is limited, and especially in a time where resources are rapidly becoming scarcer that is our first concern. In that sense people helping each other developing health also are a think-tank, a generator of new ideas and understandings in dealing with what plays now and that will play in the future. Happy health gaming then.

PART 4

Becoming a Daolander. How to make Yangsheng work for you

Introduction: Global trends in natural health care

The main topic of this book is 'how to take best care of our health'. The method we discuss is a form of what can be called 'informed self-care'. The Chinese name for this is yangsheng. Yangsheng means 'growing life', or 'nourishing and cultivation of life' because Sheng is a farmers concept. Yang relates to breeding lifestock and Sheng to growing food. It includes weeding as well as education, drilling, guiding etc. it is both protective as well as hopeful and seeking freedom to flourish in the way most suitable.

This concept of Yangsheng should not been confused with the concept of life-force as is used in western esoteric thinking. Life force as used ion western countries originates in Christian thought and therefore is something given to people by God, the 'breath of life'. In Chinese thinking we have the concept of 'life qi', not to be confused with the yangqi from yinyang, another more well-known Chinese cultural concept.

Life qi is the functionality of living. It is not a force, it is a quality marker. It is based on acquiring skills, which according to this unique Chinese view are part of our human survival heritage. The better the quality of life is, the more full time functional you would be in life, and the longer you would be able to live. In modern science the possibility of lengthening life is often measured on the amount of heartbeats one goes through. It is suggested in that science that if you slow your heartbeats you would live longer. When you live more slow (less stressed) you might live longer.

The yangsheng theory does not necessarily disagree with that, although it would also accentuate a 24/7 activeness without getting stressed. When you think that strange, think again: a stone is how much alive? Not much. Heaven moves all the time and is alive a lot. Earth moves all the time, and lives already a long time too. Yangsheng, healthcare, is therefore the science of movement. How to cultivate and nourish movement. Movement = life. No movement = no life. It is the foundation of Chinese sciences on culture, health, medicine, economy even and anything else. It is how we wish to let you and your cultural background benefit from this understanding by letting you review and re-experience what you think you know. If the book and you match well, you will enrich your science of life and become more successful in being happy, healthy and long living.

We will take a look at this heritage and give suggestions on how to make it work for you. At the same time we introduce the Daoland self-care program as a means to acquire and test the inherent skills of being a surviving healthy human being.

The ideas of Chinese culture on health

Traditional Chinese Medicine both as a historical phenomenon and as a product of post Maoist China posits a that there is uniquely relative relationship between the Wuzhang-Liufu (5 granaries and 6 factories as organs) and the tissues and tissue networks of the human body, as well as between the human body, the mind and the natural environment. From a modern perspective we could say that the Chinese approach included social theory, moral theory and biological theory in one package.

Several schools of thoughts do exist in the field of Chinese medicines, and they do give different descriptions of the relations. But in fact they do come all back to a limited set of rules to determine mechanisms. They are formulated within the Yinyang polarity theory and Wuxing consuming relationship theory mostly, but other theories have been formulated too. Altogether we may not that there are 13 theories being the most prominent ones. From these theories it is stated that all components of this tripart unity of mind, body and environment are in a relatively balanced state (homeostasis) in order to maintain the person's normal physiological, psychological and social functions. When this balance is destroyed disease results in the form of physical, mental or social distortions.

Through long term clinical practice, some ancient Chinese 'doctors' realized that there are many factors which may bring about imbalances in the human body and thus disease such as climatic abnormalities, pestilence, emotional stimulation, injury by irregular diet or overstrain, trauma, insect-bites, etc.. On top of that they also recognized that disease is not without an after effect which can by itself be a serious problem. Pathological products of disease outcome, such as blood stasis, phlegm-humor, etc. are among these. All of these contribute to imbalances within the human system.

All these manifestations differentiate the person and the person's health from the normal state of existence, the study of which is summarized in neidanxue 内丹学 internal medicine studies, yangshengxu 养生学 growing life/birthing studies, sheshengxue 摄生学 studies in gleaning life/birthing, zunshengxue 遵生学 studies in respect for rules of life/birthing, weishengxue 衛生学 studies in defense of life/

birthing. In the se the words of yangsheng and neidan are most commonly used in popular vernacular of these studies.

These study fields implement that the practice and study of healthy functioning is more important than the study of curing or treating disease. This not only because it helps one prevent the onset of debilitating disease and delay the onset of serious aging and thus lessen the impact of suffering on the quality of life. The health promoting approach as a continuous involvement with oneself in life also implies a study in personal and social morality processes which extends the study of health into the practice of religion through Daoism and Buddhism, and social politics through the study of Confucianism.

An active component of all health and disease related studies in Chinese medicine culture is the active involvement of the pursuit of the enigmatic Dao(道), often translated with 'the way, since the character for dao originally meant 'tracking/ finding your way in the wildernis'. The meaning of the concept of dao is elusive. Laozi did set the tone for medicine studies by telling that daode (道德) -morality is the 'reason d'etre' of cultivating life. He also said that Dao is amazing and maybe incomprehensible through 道可道非常道, translated as 'dao that dao's is amazing dao' or even that 'dao at work is amazing', implementing a state of wonder resulting when one perceives the perfection of dao (by means of its qi 氣 the ghostly presence of location or qi 炁 the fiery effect of the absence of thingness). Laozi also suggested that 道生一·一生二·二生三·三生万物: Dao births/grows one, one grows two, two grows three, three grows the 10000 beings. The one we talk of here is 太乙, taiyi, or the greater unity/oneness of things, that is exemplified in Buddhist unity of everything in consciousness, and Daoist unity of everything in life. Moreover, taiyi also is explained as the god that overcomes suffering that stands at the beginning of all existence. In fact when we read into modern biological science we see that neurobiology tends to see consciousness as a dream-state that is altered by sensory input to shape its beliefs or by memories when dreaming, which allows for positive assessment both of the Buddhist as well as the Daoist perception of oneness of things.

We stated that Daode-morality as part of health and disease studies is very elementary. This relates as much as to what one ought to do in life for oneself as well as for one's community. Maintaining health in mind, body and behavior is a triangle of interrelated ethical issues. But health and disease studies also relate to further connects through the study of daoyi 道義 *righteousness and daoli* 道理*-rationality/reason. In heangdineijing suwen it says that:*

In remote antiquity, the shengren 聖人 (holy man/sage) did teach his subjects how to be timely in avoiding noxious substances (邪) that appear out of season and be calm and without desire, anger and fear. Then the zhenqi 真氣-true qi will arise as of itself. If one can maintain the integrity of one's awareness (精神, construction of awareness) and control one's feelings, then how can disease come about?

So then if this is the study of health, then the study of disease then is the study of what happens when people do not hold one to the integral unity of body, mind and life.

The Daoland Yangsheng program is about people making personal choices to take a radical new direction in health management. Health management has developed many high

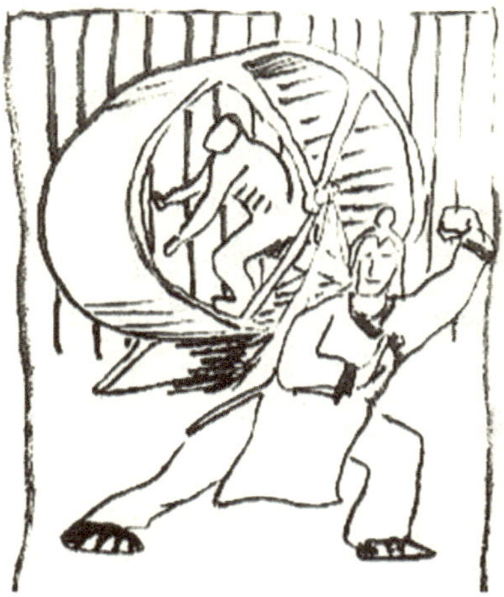

tech solutions in the last 50 years, such as the use of exercise machines, electrical impulses of the muscles to make them grow rapidly, medicines to boost performance end battle disease. It is based on developing the parts to benefit the whole.

The Daoland Yangsheng approach takes the opposite direction, which is the Low-tech approach: the Daoland program allows the user the exploration of the possibilities the mind and body offer themselves for fun, beauty, fitness and health. It is based on developing the whole by integrating its parts. With the Daoland healthcare programming and skills development we hope to make people aware that our body includes all the technology we need to be healthy and fit, take care of our looks en our intelligence as well. It is a natural technology, in contrast with artificial technology. We people are technology, developed in eons of differentiation between different life processes.

Mechanical technology often contributes to our stress levels because of one-sided singular practice. It also increased the change for trauma. Natural technology has all kinds of fail-safes build in that allow us to grow from statistical nominal health to having Life Qi, or even Gongfu. Daoland Healthcare is about developing ideal health in a natural way. Natural self-help is a good tool to find peace for oneself but as one of global unity and peace. Daoland healthcare takes care of form and content of the body, development of inner awareness and ability to influence processes, and the skill to develop pleasure in taking part in life.

The Daoland health program is the first green holist approach to health that appears in the 21st century, or maybe ever. Health programs of the past usually theorized about links with the environment, such as in Chinese medicine and sports on which Daoland is strongly based. In participation no artificial means are used and this makes participation cheap. From the professional viewpoint, investment in developing healthcare is less than a fraction of western healthcare systems, which makes it a substantial contribution in poor, rich and impoverished countries. It includes personal community building as well as personal individual development. People are seen as a piece of environment and an extension of their environment. But as far as ecology was concerned... the Chinese healthcare roots of this program offer nothing less and beyond immortality training, that is: conserving oneself to live forever.

This modern time shows that we squander our natural resources not only in industry and consumerism, but also in how we deal with ourselves. By allowing our body health to develop randomly and uncontrolled we also generate dependencies on which an extensive medicine industry booms and pollutes our environment. Our health becomes a patchwork of quick fixes that props up holes with pieces of unclear materials. For every crutch or pill or bandage the sky becomes more muddy with dirt particles, the soil more salienated with cotton fertilizers, and the water more polarized with chemicals. This pollution we have learned leads to more allergies, insufficiencies of our body organs and so on. Ofcourse there are those companies that benefit from that, and some of their chieftains themselves show great concern for the environment too, but as a whole our lack of self-care is not green. It is more like fast-food. Even though our problems can be debilitating we grab our quick-fixes in passing by, treating our body as a servant instead of realizing we are our bodies. Eating well in itself does not make us healthy. In fact if we would only eat biologically grown food there would not be enough soil to feed all the billions of people and give nature itself also lebensraum. Eating more efficient therefore is of great value to us, and for that we need to have healthy bodies that can do that. It is time that our healthcare teaches us that our intestines, our blood system, our breathing and our emotions all require practice too, not only some muscle groups. We also have to realize that different skills require different approaches to moving, that there are a variety of movement systems in the world that allow a broadening of our understanding both of health as well our capacities as people. The Daoland program is a platform that has to make this visible and usable to science and the general public. Therefore the approach of Daoland offers the following:

- *Consciously Internalized Event Awareness Guided (exercise) programs to help manage the emotive-chemical processes inherent to health maintenance*
- *Studied Internalized care and supportive programs to help develop skills in self- management*
- *Maximalized natural beauty generating programs by gradually enhancing the natural ability of the body to heal itself and generate wellbeing*
- *Dietary awareness training so as to maximize benefits from conscious eating and slow food programs*

Do not try to think complicated about this. Although there are many programs available, they are all playful programs that allow you to perceive yourself in the same way as a gaming arcade would. Under all circumstances progress will be gradual and is based on the gradually shaping understanding that the cultural mind is capable of. This allows for the natural understanding of circumstances and the most likely outcome of results over time, not immediately. For the description of the scientific pathways of this knowledge you might need encyclopedias. But on the personal level these understandings are clear and practical as well as often self-evident on hindsight. There are no other special skills or knowledge required other than the dedication to your own health. Intelligence as people usually perceive it is not required, and as seen from the perspective of health care highly overrated too. Cultural knowledge often plays on your gut level, it is intuitive in that it shows you around and makes you familiar with the process of becoming that is life. It shows that failure is part of learning too and that there is no such thing as a static outcome of a process. All outcomes are relative, imprecise and temporarily. Health is part of this chaotic realm, which in Daoism used to be called Hundun, 'muddled chaos'. It is also translated as primal chaos, because the word Hundun is associated with the presumed healthy state at the beginning of the world, which was not fixed in form, but flawless in its own way. This is why Daoland advocates health as a process, not a clearly outlined outcome. This is why the Daoland program allows practitioners to develop its own tools, as to develop the freedom to alter your health related to the needs of your personal life. A desk-worker needs another health or fitness then a dockworker!

The program itself lets you intuitively experience yourself and your processes, makes the processes visible and shows you how to alter yourself towards health over a given period of time.

This new approach suits best in the current environmental climate where moral involvement of distributers and costumers becomes a stronger issue each year. In the past the trend was always towards technological innovation and more persuasive imagery to convince people to enter the world of health, sports or beauty. Now the trend is towards shared personal experiences, and that means mixed individual and group activities that are both health promoting, entertaining and educational and include all four major grassroot level edutainment sectors: beauty, health, sports and personal development -that are accessible to anyone and allows for adaptation to personal needs and wants of demanding modern people who like to stay fit, radiate freshness and look young.

The global trend is towards theme-based approaches in providing and requiring health support, both in resorts, sports centers and health- or beauty clinics. The Daoland program combines these trends all into one harmonious formula which is possible due to the nature of classical Chinese cultural medicines and sports.

Theme based approaches to presenting and learning about health and beauty are also called Cultural styles. These styles are the new idiom for health enthusiasts. The idea of cultural styles is the effect of globalism and worldwide travelling by just about everyone on the globe. We are slowly coming to recognize that culture for instance makes you ask question and therefore decides what kind of science a people develop. Swahili science, Chinese science and European science are by nature radically different because they are different cultures.

We see this best in the discussion of health and disease. Chinese medicine has a clear idea about a healthy person, namely the immortal. It is an idea that Chinese medicine strives for to achieve.

Health is also seen as an individual achievement. Western medicine on the other hand sees health as the absence of disease. Its idea of health is based on statistical average occurrence of health states and therefore is variable over time. When general health becomes lower, the expectations for what entails health will become lower. This difference is significant. And global exchange makes it possible to know about this and to make personal choices about health and benefit from ideas from the general average.

Because we have the choice we as people car and want to choose to what ideology and culture we like to fit into, just like they do with their clothes and cars. Some do this from a historical perspective, because their family belongs to this or that culture; some from fashion perspective; some from curiosity or fascination, but other people just let influence happen. The idea from this book is that making a choice in this helps us to get more healthy because making a choice helps us develop a system of health management.

We have over the last 200 years acquired in society the ability to make personal choices that are relevant to us and that helped make us more independent from our social situations. It is the main development of the last 250 years, namely the idea of personal emancipation, which ideas were first coined by the likes of Aristotle, Zhuangzi and Kongzi.

Although poverty is going to be part of our lives for a long time to be, absolute Poverty is for more and more people no longer what determines the course of their lives. Even in Africa, that is seen for a long time as the epitaph of failed states and accumulated human misery, more and more people are uplifted towards a standard of life that allows them to worry less about food a few days from now and more about issues that also play a role in the development of healthcare plans such as Daoland offers.

Due to education we have opened our eyes to all the alternatives the world offers, so the world gradually grows towards a more unified, maybe even holistic society. Because of study and talking and writing we gradually learn to overcome our fear for the strange and unknown.

Because of this wider understanding people don't want the same old styles of healthcare being redressed to make it look modern. They are ready for the real thing, the new, the unique and the meaningful. The Daoland self-care program, like Wikipedia, Facebook, open source programming, or better even: like the internet itself, like consumer organizations and workers and trade organizations seeks to offer a wide perspective in which people can create their own sense of reality and sensibility. The Daoland self-care system is an interactive health care method that borrows from the experience with modern technology in a variety of ways. For instance it uses internet based concepts of networking, applies them and improves on them by making people aware of the fact that their healthcare is both a geographically local issue, a cultural issue, but also global issue where people can learn from the difference in experience with the same things in different cultures. Another aspect that is innovative is that it invites people to share their health experiences in the system to help each other forward and to decrease medical dependency.

Another aspect it borrows from experience with modern technology is the recognition of technological dependency and the downsides of that as well as the fact that our body and consciousness provide a technology of their own. By creating more self-conscious life styles we can do two things. First of all we become less dependent on technological support for our lives and secondly we can adapt our technology better to our needs instead of adapting ourselves all the time to technology that has been created for mere commercial purposes. We can be wise.

Transformative health technology

Daoland offers effective tools for developing health, fitness and beauty which are personality transforming too! The great thing is that everything happens in your own pace. It is a path of self-discovery as person and body, but also a possibility to overcome hindrances to lead happy lives. In general the program helps to develop a relaxed attitude to life where there is space for play and seriousness with properly balanced feelings. As such practicing elements of the Daoland program helps developing people's identity according to their own personal interests. An identity is what people wear and feel at home with. The content of this book is proof of that. It is the experience of my life path as it is of many people all over the world.

But you may ask yourself how to acquire the benefits of this Daoland program? The answer is clear. We tap into what human beings by nature are and use that to propel ourselves forward in what we can understand about modern society. Since humans are by nature hunters and gatherers, group beings, omnivores, tool makers, family builders, sensitive beings, able to make choices -and so on- it is important to systemize these abilities in our daily life, when working in the office or hunting for the latest fashion items or exercising our body or mind for health and beauty purposes. How we do that?

1. Group Based Experiences – *because learning happens fastest when we play and playing takes place between people*
2. Individual Person Based programs – *because everyone has a unique personal development everyone also has unique individual needs*
3. Holistic Approach to Health – *because you cannot solve a problem without also working on its context*

4. Theme Orientated Programming – *because a theme helps us develop a theoretical framework on which basis we can test our progres*
5. Total Freedom Impact Methodology – *because we are only healthy when we feel free to be in control*
6. Low Tech Minimal Investment Projects – *because the only instruments and tool we need for health are we our selves*

All these programs can be executed either online or onsite, although onsite allows for some extra's that online cannot do, as does online has some benefits over on site activities. The research is focussed on online participation to reach many people in many countries.

It is very western to classify elements of training this way, but the combination of aspects is rather unique and culturally mixed. In fact, because the program is so complete it becomes a new and modern culture by itself that fits in both with western and Chinese as well as other culture's attitudes. And that is the point. Most people live between cultures or in diffuse cultures quite uninformed. Thaat lack of being informed often contributes to weak health. That means their cultures are no longer pronouncedly present in their lives due to our work and technology oriented life styles. In that respect the Daoland formula works as a magnifying glass and a mirror.

When we look at the six first indicators we see that each has a particular purpose. Group based experiences for instance keep people from the isolation of their house and prevents depression and can remedy anxieties. Internet and busy workdays tempt people to hide in the safety of their home to seek rest. But physical and psychologically that might not be the healthiest solution. Being active within social interests groups on a regular basis helps keeping us young and alert.

Being part of the Daoland program some things can be done at home, but for renewal and other good experiences that make us feel involved with social movements, with betterment of the world we come to meet people and share the moment. These aspects make that Daoland becomes an extension of our home because it is natural for people to be at home in groups and have a space where we can remain an individual and work on shared ideas. The groups create room for stimulation that is required to feel happy. It is for this same reason why people go to find peace and happiness by sharing life and celebrating their ideals in other social groups. Group loyalty creates a feel-good based connection to our life, creating a faster growth and more emotional stability. Our sense of religiousness and spirituality is based on group activity. When too often alone it loses direction and makes us feel as if we walked into a swamp or against a wall. Even animals need a social environment to flourish, sparrows and roosters are like most animals in continuous cycle of communication to help develop identity (location in a system) and health (fitness to participate in a system).

Individual Person Based Programs goes steps beyond the idea of "free choice" or "to do as you please". It allows the person to take total control over their choice and grow into responsible choices in a safe educational and entertaining environment. Guidance which is both distant and near generates trust immediately after seeing someone actually listens to us. This trust is creating good report about our experiences and progress. Listening is the foundation of all communication. Often we forget to listen because we have a need for others to listen to us, either to ventilate doubt or to hear our solutions. Communication then is a matter of mutual listening that allows one to be wrong without losing mutual respect and trust. Because like rodents we are by nature quite territorial we develop identity by believing we are right or wrong. We call these developments formation of hyper-identity and denial-identity. Being frustrated is as much an egocentric issue as is being arrogant and self-confident. So that means that many psychological problems we face are based on territorial issues. To understand this makes dealing with them much more easy. We understand that much of our identity and communication is a set of communication tricks to get our way and settle boundaries or enlarge ourselves it be positive or negative. The individual programming has to help people allow more fuzzy boundaries so that reformation of their identity can take place. The result should become more balanced with good planning and monitoring.

Developing programs for mutual support and care then is a good way of monitoring and securing development of balanced personalities because it makes that we all feel our extended families continuously enriching us as we enrich them.

A Holistic Approach to Health is indicative of a long term and growing trends starting in the 1950/60's both in Europe and the northern America's. The approach invited people to think of themselves, their body, their social life and nature as one intertwined whole. In personalized health management that indicates that people do not develop parts of themselves, but develop themselves as related to their lives and the parts of their body and their understanding of the meaning and purpose of their lives. People generally find themselves having happier lives, following this approach. It also means that their daily routines and the care they receive should reflect a holist ideology and principles of durability, since on the long run these will be the hallmarks of new societies coming about in this 21 and 22 centuries.

The Daoland approach allows for a whole package lifestyle, including care, beauty, sports, slowfood, education and other aspects that fit in wonderfully well with holism. What is the personal benefit of this? logically and experientially we quickly remember its effectiveness when so many aspects are on offer that you do not need to 'rediscover fire' and 'reinvent the wheel' and do not need to go buy specialized products (that are often highly prized). The holist approach to health is based on appreciating the common and useful, while realizing the beauty and strengths of that. Daoland is therefore not a consumerism based approach but an approach that wants to empower people to take control over many of the factors that potentially cause us to suffer and develop ill health. It doesn't offer false promises with trinkets, affirmations, forcing you to have positive thoughts or involve others in some sort of power scheme. It is solely based on applying the rules nature has already set for us and putting them into a narrative context so that we may draw benefit from them. Because that is what culture does: it creates stories which we need to give our consciousness direction, develop understanding and help us make and execute decisions. Facts are not that relevant. Facts depend on context to make them useful and context is narration, storytelling. For instance: low blood pressure. You think that is good or bad? It depends on the context. For some indeed it is bad, but if you practice taijiquan then low blood pressure is a sign of success in practice. High blood pressure the same.

Choosing to fill our lives with beautiful exclusive products are signs of territorial behavior, emphasizing our difficulty in building balanced personalities. Often we buy products to call for a bingo effect. We believe that if we surround ourselves with products of health or beauty or wealth that these things rub off on us. The products are magical talismans that have to protect us against evil that might befall us. It is a form of sympathetic magic that we never really let go of, how much we study or deem ourselves rational. Ofcourse it only works in a very few real cases. In fact what it proves is that we are not rational beings, we live in a realm of consciousness that is based on evolutionary sane causes. We started out as simply formed critters in wet layers of mud on earth, in the sea and so on. We have not grown yet beyond their direct needs.

In my classes I often compare humans with starfish. We are more complex and we have bones to help us move our limbs towards our food, but we have not really evolved yet, we still share much of the same nature with starfish: we look for food and reproduction. Although we on a relative scale are social and cooperative in munching other living creatures our needs and methods have hardly changed in millions of years. They have only diversified. Likewise we do not think much. We still go about throwing things around us as garbage as do people living in small tribes in inaccessible forests. That is our history. But the products we now litter the world with are more and not so degradable.

These childish methods of survival without thinking are called 'methods of walking on crutches'. Like crutches these methods help us feel more mobile but it is only of transitory help. It produces a state of existence filled with desperation and pain, like a tree hanging on to life on the side of a cliff by only a few roots. Ofcourse in a reasonable moment when we think about these things and can acknowledge them as truth, we can also admit that that is not the way we can continue for much longer. We live in a reality of quickly deleting supplies of minerals, drinkable water, degrading air quality and so on. The intelligence we have can and should be applied consciously and with purpose and we cannot really afford not to do so. Products should be chosen on usefulness. If a product is rare it is not useful because of overprizing, unavailability and so on. It is much like standing on one leg and trying to hold balance by groping the air. Nobody living in France requires ginseng for their health. In fact in Korea people often eat ginseng salad and they are definitely not more healthy then people in France. Sales of products is based on myths. Nobody can believe that Superman will save the world when meteorites strike, so how can eating ginseng root paste, tiger ball pills, Prozac, antibioticum or iboprufen help your health? How does jewelry or rich clothing or delicate foods prevent you to age and die? Do the spirits of stones and do angels of protection really talk to us? All these methods € us into an arc of dependency pointing to ourselves but not really involving ourselves. All these methods are about delaying the inevitable that is the result of the content-meaning of how we act. Doing special things is a personality need, not a health need. It is not that they are totally without use, but they are limited in their possible success and as such anyone advocating them as a salvation is a false prophet. The salvation comes from how we deal with our day to day functioning. My shifu You Xuande follows Daoist monastic notions that eventually all health and salvation comes from developing moral behavior and consciousness. I do believe developing moral consciousness, environmentalism etc all contribute to development of health in constructive ways, but the adaptation of our behavior, inwardly and outwardly definitely is a major contributor, that is not only important, but also a major requirement to achieve lasting health management. This is why the marriage of awareness training and skill development in Daoland programming is such a major step in the development of human and inter-human independent healthcare management.

Holist programs then necessarily focus on what we can do first and mainly by ourselves and by means of using the common.

It is a fact that comes about from many different researches: when you dedicate your life to one theme and do not waver from that, it is likely that you can achieve happiness and health.

Investigations in religiosity, prayer, qigong, sports, social media and so on show that the sense of being connected to something valuable contributes to our health more than is easy to acknowledge. It is therefore that transcultural healthcare came about. It is for people to help them, develop their cultural root and building into it practices that can help understand one's roots better, but also involve one on a deeper level with what anyone knows is nominally benefitting anyway, namely movement. By associating health sports with lifelong programming within one's natural dedications it becomes part of the natural rituals we fill our life with for the benefit our peace of mind and our health. Hence also the association with computer games, theatrical/artistic expression and even tourism such as going to a theme park like Disneyworld. Healthsports Theme Oriented Programming requires focus to a central theme in everything. Indirectly the theme is you and your background. But our Daoland health directed theme Is Wudang Gongfu. The reason for this is because Wudang Daoist culture emphasizes:

- *disciplined and patient self-care,*
- *care for our fellow beings, and developing care for ourselves simultaneously*
- *development of harmonious forms of living, working and playing together,*
- *self-development and natural augmentation as a means of developing full potential*
- *uniting health and beauty in one theory and practice*
- *uniting care and sports in one theory and practice*
- *others*

In fact the theme of Wudang culture as the backbone of Daoland health programming is arbitrary. It is just that due to my own specialization the recognition what Daoland needs is most readily found in Wudang Daoist culture in one form or another, but then in its rough and unrefined form and not made accessible to simple people like ourselves. It is the rationale behind the way of thinking that is relevant in how we organize self-care. If we look at yoga alone as an alternative example to take as a theme we see that there are many different yoga exercises, varying from body postures to body part manipulations and breathing exercises. And although any such exercise can be helpful yoga has two handicaps:

1. *Yoga never steps out of the boundaries of a limited mechanical view of the body that emphasizes strength and flexibility but doesn't string the body parts together in a harmonious flow transportable to daily handling of affairs or communication*
2. *Yoga should be set out in combination with Indian Martial arts and dance to reach physical completeness, where Indian martial arts is defined by hardness and toughness and Indian dance is defined by gentleness but both are unified in their subjugating treatment of the body. Each skill by itself shows only its limitations*

Indian and Chinese culture have connected on many fronts over time, so many practices are similar or can be classified in similar ways, that is why it is easy to compare.. Very few other cultures have been so comprehensive in investigating health. Western culture has lagged behind in that respect because it never connected mind and body in a comparable way where that was seen as useful.

Many other cultures likewise. The Daoland program is designed such that it could connect with any of these cultural skills. For instance in African traditional dance styles there are moves that follow a very different body mechanics than either Indian or Chinese.

When we look at how we organize healhtcare we make in the Daoland program a conscious choice for holism. With this we refer to holism as practical, spiritual and interpersonal development.

Simultaneously we note a natural extension of Wellness and Health to provide improvement and beautification of oneself, each other and the world in a playful way. Wudang cultural style of thinking provides ideas about self-managed maintenance of human wellness and health because it integrates different cultural strains of thought. For instance, it is considered to be meaningful to emulate ones betters. What is better than emulating immortals? Immortals are the imagination of idealized human types. They are considered to move about in graceful and self-contained ways, much like bamboo in the forests, almost as if dancing and with purpose. The idea is that by imitating things you gradually become aware of how it functions. If we imitate monsters we gradually become monsters and if we imitate angels we gradually become angels. The reason is because we are creatures of habit and we have difficulty in breaking our habits. Habits provide a sense of safety and offer a foundation for person-bound happiness.

So, these ideas are not based on serving one's own management alone, but taking your direct and indirect environment into account. Each and one of us is part of our environment and a s such have an impact on it and our environment impacts us.

There is a difference between health practice in Wudang itself and that in Daoland. Daoland follows common modern ideas about personal independence and so on, even in learning. In

Wudang culture that is not always the case. Learning takes often place in a more military style where someone dictates what and when you learn. Learning is organized more random according to lines of power and need. Not so in Daoland, Daoland takes learning to be the same as play. One needs to experience some wonderment when practicing oneself. Wonderment on things helps us to investigate. Daoland also is a community. When we all care for each other, after all, we also have people actually taking care of us and caring for us. This is part of the bond between Wudang community members that call each other brothers and sisters. But here, following modern insights in social needs, and even Mozi from over 2000 years ago, that everyone needs to take care of everyone if we want to be able to handle the problems we face individually and as a species. This is no longer a time where we can allow special interest groups rule our lives or the world as a whole. We can no longer follow the non-holist approach of tribal people that we still are, that had in the past no idea of the impact of their waste and exploitation. This is such an habit to provides us a feel of safety, but in fact is damaging us. We have to learn think like one big family on a small island: by means of developing and maintain life and health we automatically become caretakers of the world too.

This simplicity is attractive because it combines the known and the exotic, the ancient and the new, the self and the world. It also gives a good reason to investigate and improve the totality of your life and health and so on. This programming is actually teaching about the importance of ordinary daily activities. This process requires only small adjustments over time without losing its attraction and usefulness. We in fact only take our behavior and bodily functions in account and do not require instruments, nor costly ingestives such as herbs or chemical medicines, hence lower long term investment needs. We simply learn how to use our bodies, breathing, feelings and digestion more effective. Once we install a holistic lifestyle of choice in fact we come to automatically raise the next holistic generation so that the effects of what we do becomes deeper rooted in the wellness of all people.

The fifth aspect is called Total Freedom Impact Methodology, which is allowing a gradual and intuitive self-discovery within the program. This way the program keeps adapting to changing needs from year to year, and therefore remains new and interesting. This is important because every 7 or 8 years or so the trend of our health nature changes.

These changes are relevant because they determine how we perceive ourselves and they allow us to work forward to what to expect and what to prevent. According to Chinese medicine observation men and women grow through notable cycles of construction and deconstruction. The first 7 or eight years of our life is called the cycle of growing yang. It means that people have an urge to grow on all levels of existence causing us to burn hot, be changeable but also not too well coordinated in thoughts, feelings and action. To support our growth we need disciplining exercise. Whenever we need to revalidate the principles are similar. When we enter the next cycle we establish our fertility. This stage we can call the flowering into life. We actually start to become persons. The next stages are stages of ripening and gradual development stability and from about 40-54 years upward our body starts winding down causing a gradual cascading of malfunctions, eventually ending in actual drying and shriveling, emptiness heat, irritability, impatience, loss of consciousness. In life cultivation programs we work on delaying that inevitable decay or creating a buffer that prevents the onset of diseases resulting from aging.

Aspect number six was in fact already mentioned in aspect number four: Low Tech Minimal Investment Project is what we get as true value for our efforts. Skills learned remain part of a lifelong package that can be elaborated on. Since we mainly use our own selves, bodies, minds, normal foods and drinks and social lives as tools, we come to adapt ourselves more consciously to higher and higher demands from an ongoing technocratic development in society at large. The idea is to implement healthcare as much as possible in normal life. So healthcare should become integral part of how we educate ourselves in the way of life. Learning ion how to handle life and health is much more important than learning a career, since a career depends on ability to handle life. This also includes learning how to eat, how to move, how to not move, sleeping and party behaviors, because also finding enjoyment in things is part of healthcare. In fact, healthcare suggests that enjoyment comes from two things:

1) relief of suffering
2) actual enjoyment.

Most people experience enjoyment to not notice their suffering and therefore their enjoyment comes from the first category. But enjoyment should come simply from being alive. Enjoyment is part of the urge to live and is not a masking of dissatisfaction

The Hierarchical Daoland diagram

Hierarchy is by many nowadays looked upon with suspicion. But like our computer programs and the stories of history hierarchy is inevitable part of our existence. Understanding hierarchy is part of understanding the Dao of health.

As explained above the Daoland approach is a neigong (internalized practice) approach to yangsheng (health cultivation), which means that attention is given to the experience of exercise as a means to induce improvements in experience and results. This is a natural feedback mechanism that does not require additional measuring devices, although the measuring devices themselves show that open minded attention is a major tool in making improvements.

Below we offer a statistic that includes the whole range from being alive to being death, which is basically the range in which our life and health take place. Usually death is being excluded from these kind of statistics, but using Chinese medicine theory as the foundation for statistical comparison including it was the logical thing to do and in fact also for people who know nothing about Chinese culture, when they stop to think about it they find it makes sense to include it too. In fact it shows how disease is a part of aging and dying. And that is in fact essential in our Daoland message. We see that life takes place between passive and active participation in our life, internal factors and external factors. The assumption here is that when we are dead we are surrendering fully to external factors and lease full control over our destiny. It is an outcome we all least prefer. It is the outcome with the largest amount of dependency, such as care is an aspect of.

When we look at the first hierarchical diagram we see that the root if the diagram is health and health cultivation. In the first diagram we see three main factors in developing health, called practice, care, internal factors and external factors. In the first model we see a worst case scenario of disease, namely being death. In that case here is some after care by the people mourning for you and missing you, or take care of your grave or being happy you no longer suffer. But the biggest part of us is external factors which merge with the internal factors and there is no self- motivated capacity at all to alter the situation, at least if for now we cancel out the opportunity of living some form of afterlife. It also shows health is dependent on how much we take ourselves by the hand and not on how much we rely on being taken by the hand by people who have an economic interest in us not being too well.

When we are sick we are driven by our disease. External factors and internal factors go rampant with us and we are in great need of care. So we have lost independent existence. In a healthy situation we see that practice of exercise and health more or less even out the internal and external factors. We see that being sick and aging takes as much time investment as being healthy. Being sick and doing the aging thing makes us lose valuable time. Especially because it brings down the quality of the time we have left. We need that time to recuperate. When we did spend this time on being healthy the quality time left is of a much higher level and therefore we enjoy life much more. therefore when we consciously investigate ourselves and commit ourselves to health cultivation we see that gradually practicing oneself reduces the need for care but also diminishes impact of internal and external factors.

What it comes down to is that yangsheng (healthcare) does not require herbs or good habits alone, but a conscious management of life, and that exercise is the basis of learning, managing and developing health and long happy lives. Anybody having studied Chinese medicine thinkers from the past knows that many of them applied exercise as part of what they tried to show to people about health: Huangdi, Shennong, Peng zhe, Laozi, Zhuangzi, Hua Tou, Sun Simiao, He Gong, Tao Hongjing, Chen Tuan, Zhang Sanfeng, Li shizhen to mention just a few names every Chinese medicine practitioner knows about. Exercise is a form of practicing healthy identity and preparation for future moments of crisis as well as dispersions of tensions and pollution resulting from old moments of crisis.

Does Daoland healthcare then aim to eliminate medicine all together? No it is not. It is based on the responsibility we have to ourselves to avoid spending millions on healthcare, making insurance companies rich in the process when all that is not necessary. Medicine should be applied only in situations healthcare cannot handle by means of keeping ourselves healthy. The money could also be spend on education, cleaning up environmental pollution, other useful issues that now lack attention.

The interesting approach of Daoland Healthcare is that is shows that proper practice of one's mind and body also provides a safe preparation for medication and other care generating activities when they are indeed required to solve the acuteness of a medical or psychological issue, minimizing side effects, pollution and other forms of harm resulting from taking herbs or chemicals to support recovery from a problem. So we are here not talking about complicated internal manipulations to solve problems by means of meditation and internal gazing, but simply that being actively involved in receiving care and giving oneself care as if one is exercising will do three major things:

1) *it reduces the negative impact of poisonous side effects of medicines and other high impact procedures*
2) *people can do with lower doses of medicine since the body is more quick to respond on influence*
3) *it requires less intensive care procedures to maximize the effect and therefore allows for higher sensitivity development in care providers.*

Both beneficial factors result in better and faster results in most procedures, but ofcourse also require clients and care providers to have similar understandings about health. The information spread through the Daoland courses and other publicizing media does exactly that.

Below we find the second diagram, called the Health/ Yangsheng diagram that includes all exercise systems of the Daoland program and subdivides them into care and sports. Care programs stimulate sharing and mutual cooperation and communication. Sports allow one to investigate oneself in preparation for care or development of health. The main theme in all these activities is to develop rejuvenation: retrieving youthfulnes, or what in Daoism is called 'returning to ones origin' and the revival of yuanqi or vitality.

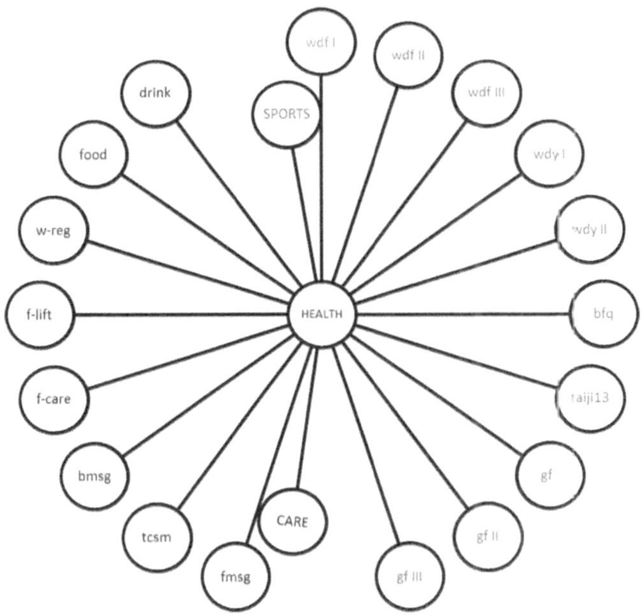

Earlyer version of the daoland diagram based on the yinyang partition of doing things yourself and being taken care of

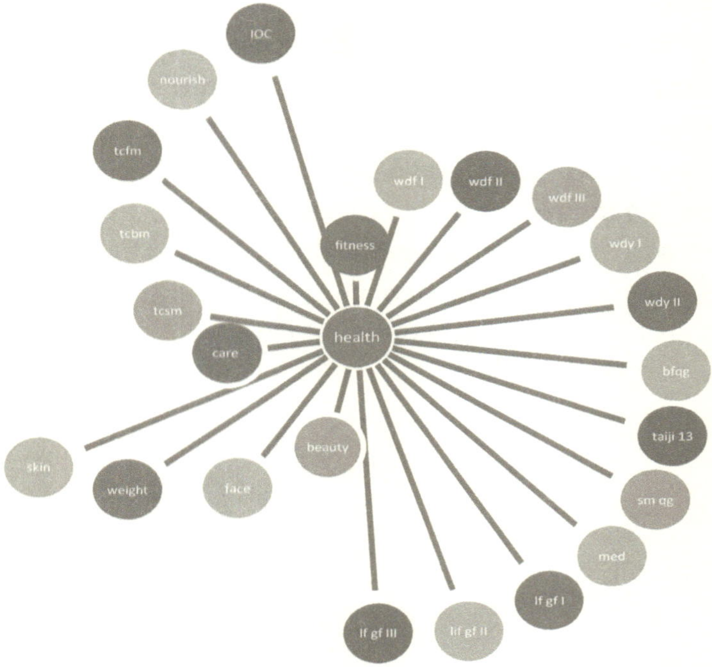

Current version of the Daoland diagram, revealing the tripart interaction between Exercise, Beauty and Care

There are three groups of activity in the Daoland program. Firstly there are the health sports, then there is the theoretical cultural education plan, third is the care program. For each of these the instructors require specialized programs to be able to implement the whole of the Daoland idea in their daily work. When entered into the program the participants usually find that it allows plenty for experiment and personal development.

Rejuvenating health sports

The first group we will shortly discuss belong to Group-sports and Individual Sports. I mean with this that people learn the skills in shared time with other people, who all might be of different levels and therefore can serve as a wonderful set of references. At the same time each participant him or herself remain conscious that he or she self is the one who is learning and practicing and therefore keep track of her or his changes wherever they take place. For most people keeping notes in a notebook -like a health diary- allows one quickly to track positive and negative changes and therefore to direct one's progress much faster. But primarily we have developed the following set of courses:

- Wudang fitness I, II, II for developing leg based balance, flexibility, strength, playfulness, spatial intelligence, patience, endurance, vegetative body control, stress control, natural breathing, general wellbeing and calm. Wudang fitness is developed out of practice trends in taiji gongfu warm op play, called xing gong. Xinggong means 'improving ones form'. We may call it body shape practice. When we use the force of the pressure we offer the earth when standing consciously we generate what is called Earth Qi. In contrast with the name, earth qi is caused because its ability to resist our consciousness and weight force to sink back into the earth. Is such Earth Qi is comparable with the reactive forcer as used in physics, except that in Daoist skills its subjective nature as and experience is used to produce force, and not the measurable body weight alone. In this sense we see that this ancient way of thinking produces science on different grounds than instrumental science from the west has done.

  This force is guided upwards in the body to become strength and the particular style of movement people often associate with water-like, snake-like and crane-like movements. What is called the muscle channels guide them along particular pathways and their strength and ability nourishes the quality aspects of our body, which is called body-yin. For most people this force will accumulate in the head and thus cause aging and dizziness, fuzziness, slowness and so forth. The point is to learn divert it to the arms and restore the possible harmony of our body structure.

Wudang fitness I is helping one to develop agility and increased body balance, endurance and speed. It does so by regulating the breath during speedily performed qigong baser aerobic practice. The breath regulation helps one to understand the spaciousness of the body and our feelings under stress. When we stress ourselves our body becomes dark and desperate. The practice allows one to move in the opposite way and maintain our sense of openness and brightness. Due to the fact the sessions are not guided by music our movements do not become uniform, but remain organic. You learn to appreciate the rhythms of your own body, to develop at your own speed beyond the levels that practice guided by music would allow for.

In Wudang fitness II the form of movement is practiced by means of particular slow movements, though which one's strength, internal coordination and balance are improved. Both practice systems are charged with many exercises allowing for gradual increased complexity in cultivation programs, keeping participating interesting and challenging. Also this practice goes without musical accompaniment. It takes development of mental focus and spatial coordination and the limbic system of the brain as its root. It also increases blood production and contributes to strengthening our bones while keeping them flexible. Usually practice goes through different stages: hardship, clumsiness and developing grace and enjoyment. The reason for this is because people try to force themselves to be strong. You do not need to force yourself to be strong, you need to become smart and find out where strength comes from and how it is guided.

Wudang fitness III originates in zhan zhuang (standing like a pole) practice from wudang pai. It is also closely related to the new sport of planking, which is also included in some advanced exercises. Usually I advise students to combine this one with food and drink training to prevent them to develop gaining weight, but in itself this practice is a great help in developing joint and movement. In standing like a pole one increases ones daring to relax under stress. You also realign the position of joints, nerves and muscles to offer greater resilience. It improves muscle and bone strength and it allow for development of kindness and patience, micro-coordination and -awareness. It is a set of thirteen practices of increasing difficulty combined with a softening qigong.

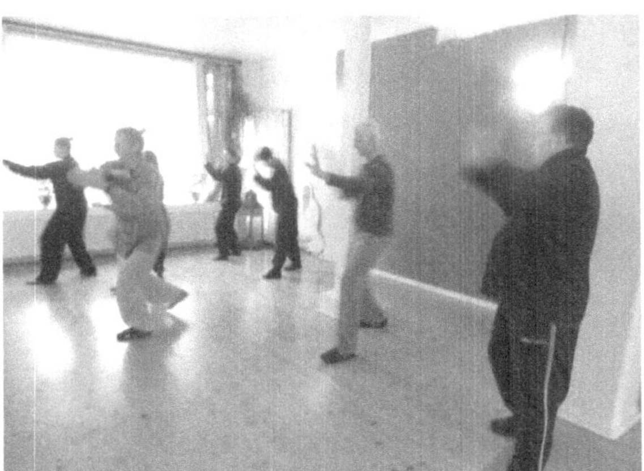
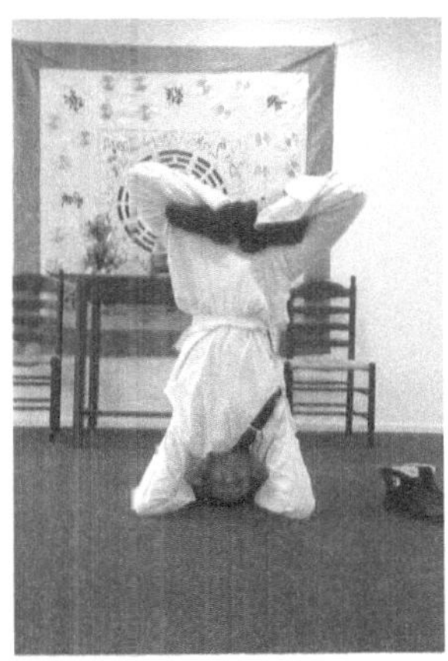

In all these three classes the legs are the roots of strength and flexibility, following the Zhang Sanfeng saying that "force originates in the legs/feet, is coordinated within the waist and expressed in the arms/palms". These three groups of exercises help one to remain vital and mobile well into ripe age. They also help us remind that moving in itself is helping to prove one to be alive, but that healthy movement creates life. Classes are set in simple programs of one hour each in which variation, the unexpected and playfulness are combined with a silent environment. Mostly when people do exercise they do this based and rhythms from background music. The root cause for this is that army practice usually involves masses of people that need to be coordinated to quickly notice deviations in form by single instructors. When one practices with headphones this is not the case, but one isolates from the environment and drifts of in a secondary level of awareness, where the experience of the body is only partly noticed. In Wudang fitness the individual results of practice is based on the experience of one's own natural needs and rhythms so as to make progress in a natural way, almost as if one is standing on Wudang mountain itself, in the comfortable breeze of one's own awareness. People who practice these classes for some time find often that when people who come from common sport programs cannot keep up with them while they themselves do not feel as if they put much effort in their program. Practicing this way is very non-competitive but allows one to gradually up one's standard on the basis of experience of convenience and ability.

- Wudang Daoyin/Yoga I, II for developing arm based balance, flexibility, strength, spinal openness, concentration,

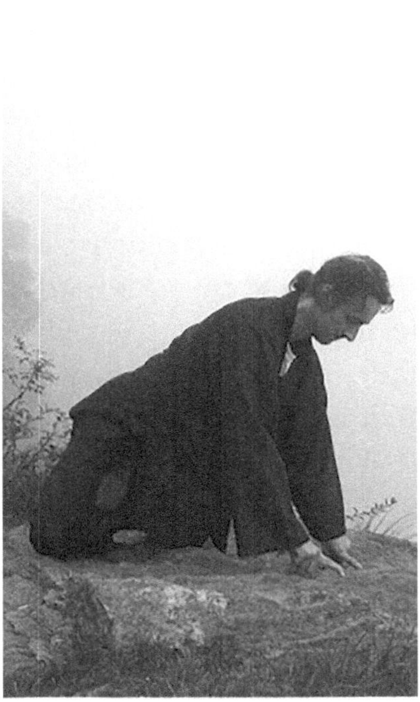

inner sensitivity, patience, endurance, vegetative body control, stress control, power breathing, general wellbeing and smiling attitude. In fact these are simple breathing practices to help one develop a better lung-kidney connection, which is the foundation for breathing according to Chinese medicine study. It is specific Wudang practice for strengthening dantian and the development of yuanqi, yang and yin. The process of breathing is developed into two directions and are mildly stimulating the body to develop inner and outer flexibility and strength coordination through the coordination of strength, breathing and directed concentration. Daoyin is a the original Chinese word for yogic practices in which experiences are guided by pulling and pushing internal substances. It is a foundational skill in all Chinese yangsheng practice. Wudang yoga helps increase the effectiveness of other skills enormously. Wudang Yoga is different from Wudang fitness because it is based on fixed sets of exercise that also follow a fixed order outside the period where one is learning the exercises. It is though similar like Wudang Fitness that effect is gained though practicing whole sets and not its individual parts alone.

Wudang Yoga I works towards exquisite hand strength and relaxation by means of breathing. In the practice you use the breath to brighten up the tensions in your

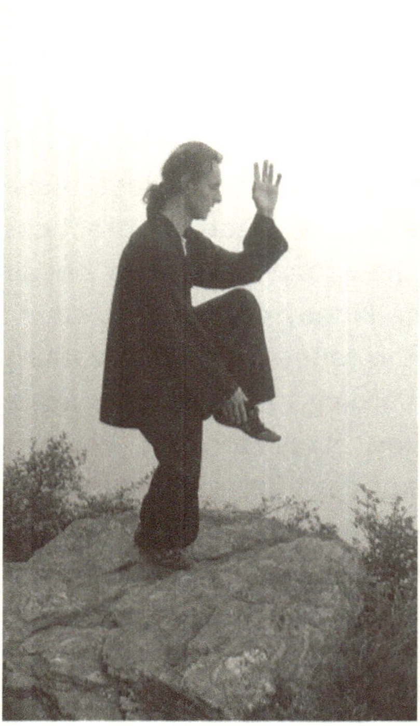

deepest body cavities. In doaist practices this belongs also to the group of practices that are called untying of karmic knots. These deep lying myofascial hardenings cause much more limitations and clumsiness in life than people realize. It gradually grinds our personality in something based on subliminal awareness of not being able to accomplish anything in an easy way or only partially accomplish things. One is than left with a lingering dissatisfaction with things that one cannot solve. Wudang Yoga I also helps one to use one's inner breath to fill ones muscles to develop above normal strength without excessive muscle formation. Like Wudang fitness one it shows economic ways of providing the muscles with fuel and getting rid of the poisons so that we do not need to worry about all kind of limitations build in by the way people slave their body with in regular sports. Wudang Yoga II follows on Wudang yoga I. This second direction helps one to develop inner awareness, allowing for awareness of inner processes on any scale, to help one guide one's health cultivation process. The origin of the classes is based on the principle of preparation of preservation of one's consciousness before dying by sealing the sense organ exits. It applies a variety of forms of breathing and circulation in which experts can recognize the small heavenly circulation (micro cosmic orbit) and the breathing and substance circulation of

Naropa which became famous in Tibetan Buddhism. The combination is very complete as an experience and forms the basis of the Wudang Yoga II daoyin set. Although it starts with very deep concentration practices for which also proper hand strength is required, but it guides one back from this deep intensity to quietude and normalcy. That is also its purpose: to connect the spiritual and the mundane in one unified whole by means of producing and regulating yang, meaning body warmth and improved circulation in this context.. The classes are set in carefully timed sequences to help fit in busy city life agenda's without losing their effectiveness. The classes last one and a half hour because the mind and body need time to develop oneself during the exercises. The mind alters usually more slow. The purpose is that the mind finds a cool balance where one feels elevated and clear minded. The slow guided breathing and the internal softening process help one to balance out physical stresses that normally stay hidden. Outwardly the body is using itself as a group of levers and pullies to address the many muscular groups required for building strong bodies.

Although music can be present in a class like this, I try myself to avoid it because music too easily sets the tone for a nature of our consciousness that is not the result of practice but of the composer and musician. It is easy to become susceptible to influences when you relax, but when practicing or in daily life we too often find that we are the result of our outside influences and not of our self-producing processes.

- Wudang Taiji 13 form practice for developing asymmetrical body intelligence, spatial intelligence, concentration, fine motor skills, creative thinking, communication skills,

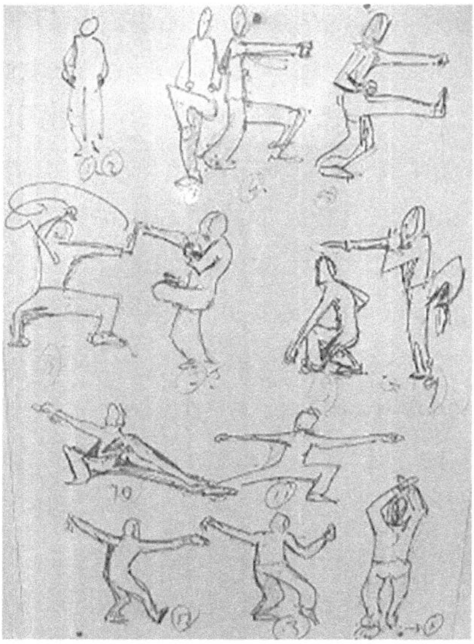

stress guidance, overcoming blood and bone related issues of weakness, preventing aging. This form has a limited set of movements which makes it easy to learn and to quickly absorb the benefits of taijiquan practice. The purpose of the practice is to help yourself develop sense of and control over the eight bodily directions as resulting from the five steps. The classes are systematically short in sessions of only half an hour dedicated form practice and alternate with a following half hour of xinggong practice of principles. These basic practices are helping one to investigate the movements used in the form so that the form itself becomes sort of a storage device helping to develop our physical capacity to stimulate our own health.it is a function that we also require in daily life, but that most people are not able to acces so that repeated efforts are made to reinvent movements on a regular basis without ever mastering them or improving on them. The classes can have background music, but like in the fitness they easily dictate the rhythm of the moves. In taijiquan practice the movement usually starts being learned slow, but over time the jing-constructive and shen-awareness of the body become a driving force that allow for natural speeding up without losing jin-power and li-strength. That process does not take place if one ritualizes class practice without taking into account one's feeling relationship with what one does. These words all sound complicated, but they are cultural concepts that help one understand one's own language much better by trying to avoid replacing them with an inappropriate term from your own cultural background. In that sense the language of the themed classes help one re-appreciate one's origins very much. This in turn benefits health a lot.

- Wudang Longform boxing wushu basics I,II, III for developing muscle control and muscle strength, developing acuteness in attitude, concentration, endurance, pride, discipline, independence. Proper meditative training is nowhere without the ability to also mentally focus under duress. Wushu is the perfect counterbalance with taiji based sports because it enhances li- muscle strength. Practice is very straight forward. Taiji and wushu sports start in practice with other attitudes about learning trajectory and results. Wushu is more focused to short term results. That is also why wushu is better for children sports then taijiquan or yoga, and why wushu practice prevents complacency in relaxation in adults when practicing internalizing sports. Wushu sports is also a form of allowing yourself to be drilled and driven by circumstances. Eventually the goal is to find relaxation and roundness in moves just as in taijiquan practice. As such it is not identical in application to common wushu practice. Competitiveness is for instance not eliminated, but more a means than a goal. The first level is a short form combined with conditioning exercises that can serve as a fitness class in itself and help one just like wudang fitness and taijiquan prepare oneself for daily hardships by means of the combat oriented imagination required of the practitioner. The second and third level are increased in length and complexity and therefore increasingly function endurance and character strengthening.

- Bambooformula Qigong for developing gentle openness, grace, flexible attitude, softness, kindness, revitalization of aged and emotional processes, awareness, fine motor control, increase circulation of limbs and internal organs. This qigong is developed out of the Confucian image of the perfect gentleman with his erect and graceful body that never seems to have to make an effort in being strong but pliant. The 9 simple movements are 9 times repeated and together they are one single exercise. The individual movements are relative meaningless. They are simplified forms of zhong wuji daoyin practice, where the individual exercise does mean a lot due to the story behind each practice. The full series of the bamboo formula (meaning the bamboo solution) helps the body to open outward and therefore supports re-allocation of tensions build up in daily life. This in itself helps one to easily revitalize. I often advice bamboo formula qigong as a beneficial regeneration method for instance during -or after- chronic disease and degenerative ailments. But I found over time that people who feel somewhat insecure about their sports-like abilities or people who suffer quite a lot of stress due to relationship or work circumstances also quickly redevelop pliant minds and sensitive feelings as well as revitalized libido or pleasure in life. I first thought it would be good to help elderly people to regenerate, but many young people are already so off track in their health that the balancing act of the bamboo formula helps them step up the quality of their life too. The classes could be practiced with relaxing music since the form is constant in its rhythm during a one hour session which is every time the same, and allows for deepening of one's experience and sensitivity within the practice while gradually adjusting to its general requirements.

The alternation of movements makes it just possible to experience some light hardship while also experiencing the ability to overcome this light hardship with some ease and comfort. Very quickly elder people and people suffering degenerative diseases notice their balance increasing due to relearning verticality and therefore also doing less falling or stumbling into things. That really is a significant boost of pleasure in life.

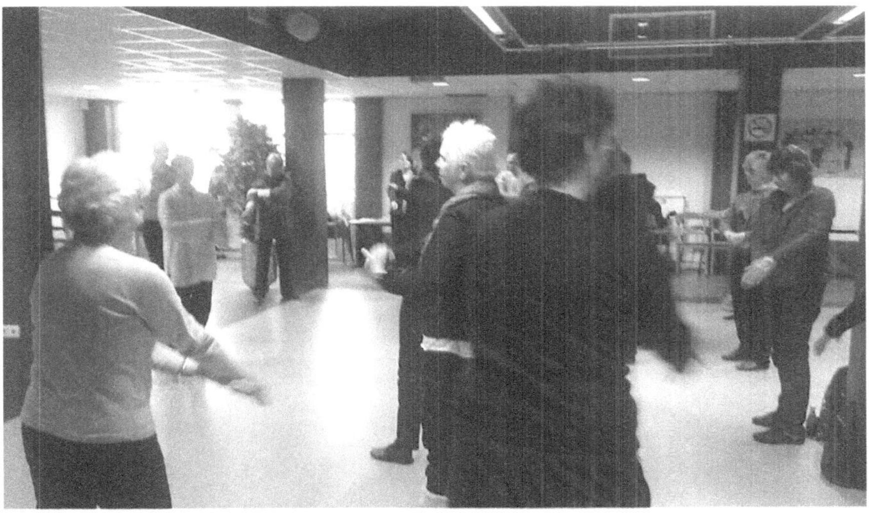

- Liu An's Selfmassage Qigong for developing self-appreciation, flexibility, increased circulation, rejuvenation of total body skin and internal organs. Self massage here points to simple dynamic movements as the drive of massaging oneself in a variety of ways, including rubbing, tapping, pulling, pressing and so on. Massaging the superficial structure of the body, face and head with the purpose of stimulating the internal tissues and organs as well as our character and self- appreciation is in itself a support for health. I learned this massage from my first major teacher Liu An, and have been refining the skills over twenty years to understand why he always suggested the importance of this practice. This self-massage applies taiji neigong principles of movement and yang development in three different overlapping sets that place ancient self-massage advices in a different and clearly also dynamic modern setting. I am still surprised how the practice keeps contributing to whole body skin maintenance, how it integrates with the Wudang fitness and yoga too. How it helps to stay warm and comfortable in the winter and cool and fresh in the summer.

Because we move during the self-massage the circulation and skin quality is additionally improved from deep within the body, where the moistness and temperature have to come from. It also offers deeper understanding of our body form and movement abilities and how they could be developed due to the investigative nature of how the movements are practiced. At the same time the self-perception is meditative allowing us to notice subtle changes and feelings and to gradually conquer our inner world as an enriched experience of life taking place. Soft background music is permitted in these classes but not necessarily supportive.

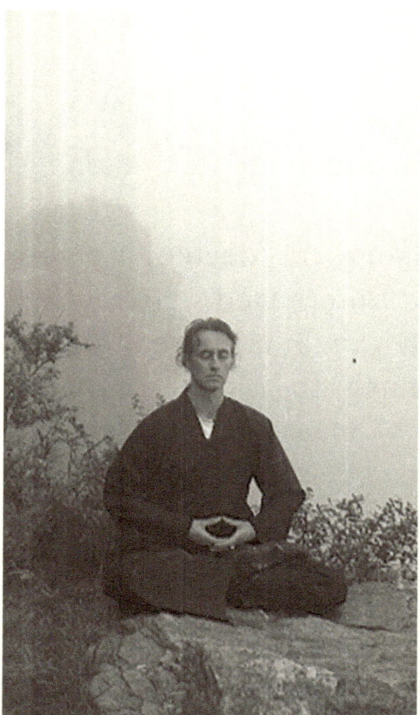

- Meditation is a sport of both the body and the mind and requires much more effort than people usually realize. People have experimented in the last century with meditation methodology because of the interaction with aspects of different cultures. Now we know meditation is a main aspect in cultural development and moral training around the globe. But meditation is also a physical achievement because one wills oneself to sit long time without moving. Different cultures meditate in different ways and with different purposes. In the Daoland meditation training we play with different basic mind states that people come across when meditating and they are related to general meditation histories and Daoism, Buddhism and Confucianism in particular. In this way the general meditation experience is outlined and one is ready to embark on a real meditation path.

Rejuvenating Wellness/Care

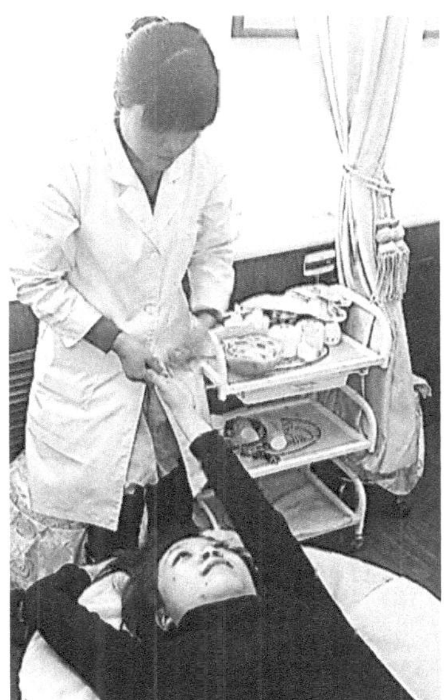

This second grouping revolves around 'being taken care of'. The point of the Daoland program is to participate in every care aspect in such a way that you yourself can increase the effectiveness of care activities. All though the Daoland is not a medical program, we see that most sub-health problems are this way easily resolved and many chronic conditions quickly find relief. The activity part is twofold. First of all you actively carry your body and use your sense organs to follow and guide the effects of the treatment and the behavior of the care giver. This is a learning process. Your active participation helps you to quickly retrieve the sensation in moments when you need it. Likewise participating in bad experiences also helps you finding wrong solutions when you need good ones. Therefore part of the care is found in the second aspect. In this part the care is substantiated as a form of dialogue, of communication. The care giver continuously provides information about what she or he is going to do or doing and asks you for your experience. If you frequently return gradually you become the mind of the care offering person, since you come to know your body experience so well. Sometimes she or he might offer you clues to what are beneficial experiences to look for. You as receiver respond likewise by offering insight in what you experience. This allows also the mind to be trained with information about rightness and wrongness in expectations and experience. For instance, when people go to Chinese massage they commonly expect forceful squeezing and pounding. First of all many masseurs have hardly received massage education so they do not understand either health or the body. Secondly, in the past people were often thickly dressed so the pounding and forceful treatment was required to get through the layers of clothing. Nowadays that is not a need but the techniques are not adapted to that, so the question is if the methods still can be considered healthy on the long run. The point of proper care is that to do as much yourself as you can and just use the care giver to facilitate change. That is application of taiji principles too. It requires specialized training of the care giver to act this way and that is what is offered in the Daoland program following the Dao of the Daoist Medicine King Sun Simiao.

- General health-boost treatment. This treatment follows a simple one point needle formula that allows for general health promotion in the same way how you take food supplements. It is not a medical intervention but a preparatory adjustment for the new season when it is arriving. A general assessment of your health is being made if you do not require therapeutic help because of your health being to impoverished (xu) or to opulent (shi). Then you are being prepped to enhance your ability to participate as much as possible in the treatment before needles are being inserted according to a standardized formula and method. Although acupuncture needles and points are being used, the treatment is based on the principles of food supplement ingestion according to western wellness ideology. In this a single treatment also cannot be effective, but a course of 10 times or multiple courses are. The effectiveness shows itself in generally increased metabolic effectiveness, improved sleeping behavior, digestion, breathing patterns etcetera. As such it can be a valuable addition to beginning yangsheng participants. It can also be advised as protection against autumn and winter weather influences. General healthboosts are best combined with the same Wudang Gongfu Fitness we use in the research. I also always advise to refrain from heating in the house if the weather does not get under 10 degrees Celcius/50 degrees farenheit.

- Acupuncture Facelifting and beauty enhancement to help people regain youthful vigor and boost their health in one package. This also is a health supporting treatment and not a medical treatment. It builds on the natural presence of yang (life) in the body, cultivates this and redirects it to the whole body, including surface tissues of your face and internal organs. In aging we normally wither like fruits in a fruit-bowl from the surface to the core. Because of this treatment method of natural aging the natural wrinkling and drying pattern of all your surface tissues as the result of aging is being battled. If dry for a long time, the wrinkles become scars, so also that issue is being addressed in the treatment with many tiny needles and according to a variety of methods. It also helps smooth blood flow as medium for moist and chemical dispersion. The result is a reduction of what we call physical aging because the body and the face become more ageless, restful and lively. The treatment also restores natural symmetries and enhances resistance against allergens and pollutions. Many other minor ailments are similarly being addressed and might melt away. The treatment is combined with specific facial and body massage, and qigong to enhance the circulation of blood. Particular breathwork can enhance the production of stem cells, which are required to speed up the rejuvenation process. For people studying Chinese medicine we use this group of practices to master yang in treatment. Yang we can call vitality.

- Acupuncture Weight Regulation to help people develop an ideal body shape and boost their health. Like the facial and health boost it is a restoring treatment which is aimed at reconnecting the natural flow between channels and intestines. It works using an ancient Chinese treatment method and improving on that on the basis of understanding more about what fatty tissue is than people did in the past. Therefore it treats also locally as well as functionally. By emptying the bowels and tightening the surface tissues gradually a process of elimination and recirculation of substances is being generated. Where in the facial yang is being strengthened here the yang is being unblocked with the result of losing superfluous weight and restoring self- confidence and enjoyable self-experience, generating a more healthy dietary lifestyle, that incorporates daily breathing exercises and wudang yoga I and fitness II too. The program works by installing improved metabolic habits and weakening the bodies bondage in its degeneration. I find this method important due to the fact that a good Antillian friend of mine died due to overweight. He was a healthcare inspector who had the worst health possible. As a result of not understanding health, health inspectors check procedures and not their actual effects. It is the worst corruption of a system possible to install fixed procedures, it is counterproductive to understanding and generating health. The Gongfu fitness can be helpfull too. Breathwork is helpful, because research has in the last few yearts shown that much overweight is lost through deep outbreathing. Also other breathing techniques are supportive. Food medicine is extremely helpful in this, becasue it advocates reducing food quantity and specific attention to the qualities we experience when eating the things we eat

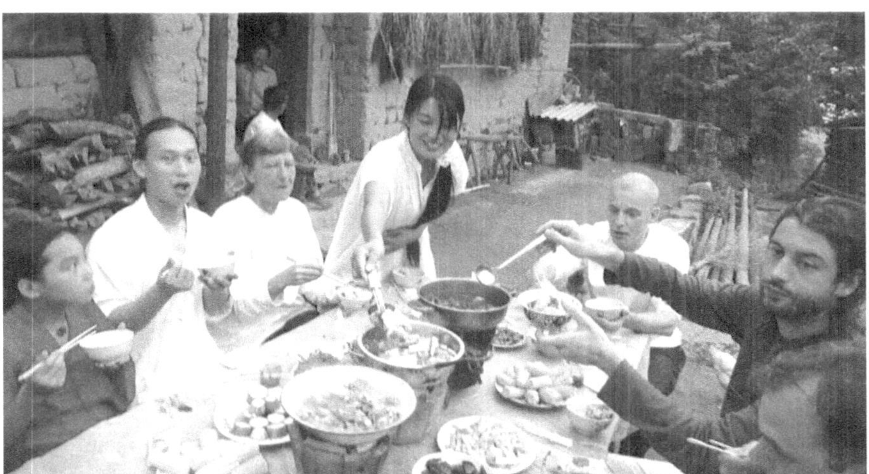

- Health supportive Food and Drink education, to enjoy healthy food and drinks to help understand how to enhance the quality of eating and drinking to benefit health and happiness. Diet in the Chinese medicine system belongs to macrobiotic lifestyle activity. It is not strictly vegetarian, but people are being made aware of the impact of food and drink on their body by directed eating drills. They learn to assess their needs for foods and as such learn that their body does not require much food but their minds because of their convictions. Because of this enhanced food awareness people tend not only to eat less, without feeling uncomfortable, but also choose less meat and fish when there is no immediate physical need for substances we cannot find in plant based diets. People are also made to experience food quality which helps to select foods for eating on a more rational basis.

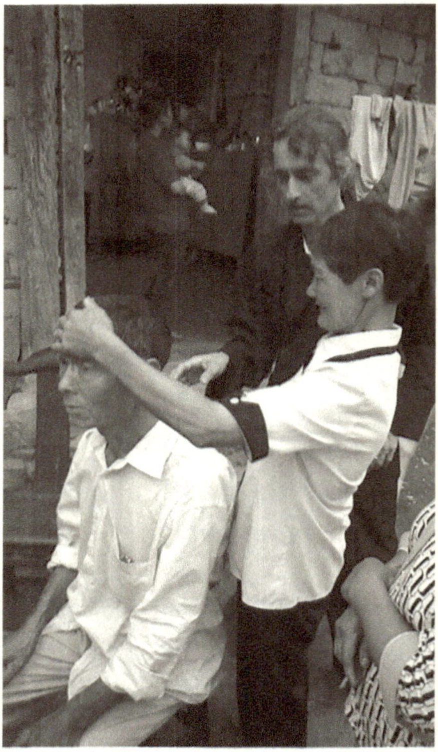

- Non-Invasive Health Massage to help people become more interactive in the support of body-mind wellness and to generally make them feel good and safe. Chinese massage has branched out in Vietnamese and Thai massage on the one side and Japanese massage on the other side. The common method in China nowadays is based on northern styles, where in the winter it is cold and the application of massage required forceful pounding to reach through layers of clothing. Western massage has branched out to sports-massage and sensual massage. They all require a level of pacification of the subject that is massaged and thus of territorial invasiveness of manipulation techniques when the massage takes place.

Non-Invasive dynamic massage styles within Daoland use the best of sensitivities developed in a diversity of massage styles from east and west and found that the ancient Chinese medicine textbooks describe massage exactly as it is being practiced in Daoland. Like all the care programs it applies Tajii principles in developing a health effect in the massage. Contrary to what people believe the single hand manipulation in massage does not have much effect, but the grouping as a whole can have this. A good massage makes you more sensitive for environmental influence to help you prevent recurring of your problems. That is why Daoland massages always are an interaction between masseur and massaged person to help stimulate awareness of natural body functions. In that way we can see Massage as a natural extension of sports programs, what it should be according to ancient Chinese medical literature. Massage bridges and prevents medical treatment. Like exercise, massage is an indispensable element in every Chinese medicine treatment to help disperse and circulate for instance needle effect and herbal infusion effects.

Massage focusing on stretching myofascial tissues, rolling and shaking to generate warmth, movement to generate circulation and patting, tapping, rubbing and so on to facilitate these actions further

- Green environment training. In Daoland it is natural to be made aware of what we can do in our environment to contribute to fortified ecological safety. Learning where we can lower our carbon footprint in our direct environment by reducing water waste, proper planting of greens that help reduce air pollution and molds, guiding our interior in other ways to help us feel home in our environment and Kings and Queens in our own country. It will take another book to go in depth on this topic. So I will leave it here for now.

- Daoland citizen care programs to create mutual support groups out of Daoland citizens in every aspect of life. We stimulate natural co-operations on voluntary basis within the Daoland precincts, but also within our daily surrounding. Opening or closing doors for peoples arriving after you or before you, helping people carrying things that are obviously to heavy, taking people out for a walk when they cannot walk very well, cooking for the poor and restoring decrepit public structures are all part of such programs. Developing education and foster homes for children without parents or housing, but elegant garden style housing and restoration of nature projects as well. You see that the original program already foreshadwoed this book and the research program I write it for.

Daoland Culture Based Science Education

There are people who just like or need to be healthy, but no health program works without health workers. The problem of being human is that learning still happens by means of example.

Intellectually we can learn a lot online, and in fact intellectual learning is a big part of becoming human, there is no denying that. But on the health level our minds just get only a part of what takes place within the body, so we need people to help us move in the right way to complement our ideas. How health practices work for someone living in culture A or in culture B maybe is not the same. If this is indeed so, the prupose of the program is to make this visible. We like to show how learning about different cultures contributes to health development and this way also generates appreciation for fellow beings in far away countries. Talking bad about people is bad social healthcare, just as it is unhealthy to not let people celebrate their own culture. Our wealth provides good education and sharing between people, so that the natural wisdom within every culture can become prevalent and paranoia or suspicions caused by ignorance and causing radicalization in east, west, north or south can be neutralized. The continuous worry bad news causes in our lives keeps the stress providing background radiation nourishing our unhappiness.

These people are our best friends in life. But we don't know them. So for some people their strengths in health feel more clear when they also help other people to become healthy.

For these and all other people we developed the instructor program, where basic skills are learned on a grass-root level to first learn get yourself in order, then your family and then the world. In the end we are all the king of our own life. The style of your self-rulership reflects in your health.

This grass-root level copies the barefoot doctor plan from the Chinese cultural revolution. In fact the idea of sending people out to solve emergency health problems is a sound idea. In Daoland we give way to our own love for our fellow beings and send ourselves in the world on the basis of the Daoland healthcare materials that also take local circumstances and knowledge systems in consideration.

Science and culture education are cornerstones of harmonious societies. Nobody can do without education and self-education or re-education. The world is changing so fast that yesterday's truths easily become today's follies. To be happy and successful in life we need to continuously grow and deepen our understanding or our self and our environment. That is also why the Daoland grass- root instructor courses take this adaptability as their root. In fact, some of the programs follow quite strict orderings of exercises and others are playful and variable. It is we who have to learn adaptation, not the exercises. Anyone adjusting methods for convenience can conclude is afraid of change and improvement. In this time many people change methods because of self-assumed insights through a presumed brilliance or high developed intuition. Although such people exist, we usually never get to know these people because they are extremely rare. We have to do with trusting in our own ability to grow. Existing exercise reflect the different needs from which learners require to receive and accept materials. Learning in that sense has to be without depth, so Daoland offers the following:

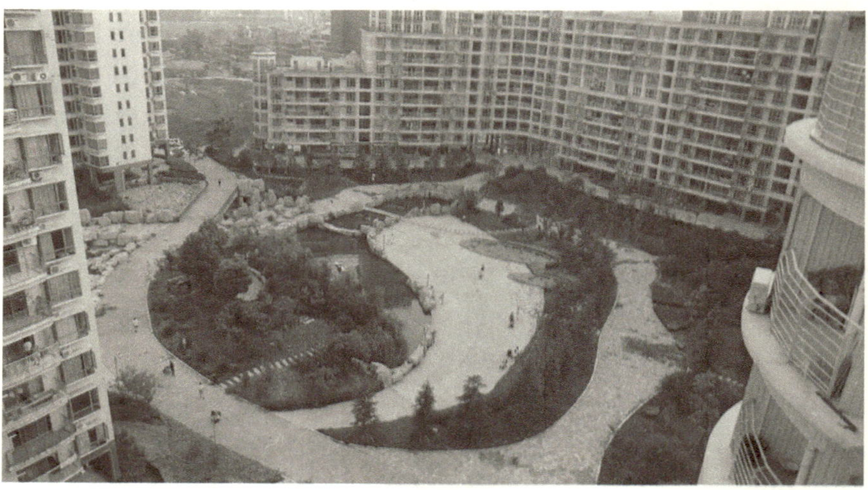

- 18 Fasttrack Instructor and Care Giving Courses as a foundation. These courses are sport and care programs following the programs above. Contributing in personal healthcare is not something for governments but of peoples themselves, that is us. Even if you will not employ yourself as such it can be handy to get insight into so many small details about how we function in a systemized way and as an addition to our regular group activities.

- Open source learning for Daoland citizens as continuous self-education program that can provide certificates valuable to career and personal life development. Vocational training is nowadays highly regarded in society. Everybody develops insights and utilizing these as a source for our success is an important element of these kind of courses. They also learn us to deal with multi-cultural contexts which are elementary aspects of developing modern societies.

- How to become Daoland official, Career training for people who would change from costumer to facilitator at any level. These are indoor programs for people who choose a career in Daoland. These courses deal for instance with how to bridge the invisible boundary between lay and professional health cultivation, how to organize work, how to deal with staff etc.

- Daoland lifestyle training for Daoland Citizens to help them engage in developing the world as a safe and healthy environment

The above diagram and explanation expresses the core activity services the Yaoland yangsheng learning program offers and how they all relate back to health for the user. 10+ services are

Wudang sports related activities, 8 services are Wudang care giving related services. The activities are larded with cultural learning to help people adjust to social requirements that can affect our health.

PART 5

Daoland's art and science of becoming a professional human

Introduction

This book is about what you can do about being healthy and not being healthy, about how the one condition changes in the other by means of our conscious and unconscious efforts. This book basically states that every second of the day we are involved in constructing health or breaking it down.

As you may well know, health is a basic human right that the World Health Organization sees as a priority in arranging human affairs. In effect health precludes much of our daily affairs because it defines us in being hopeful, desperate, moody or cheerful, hysterical or calm.

This book then is about being human.

From thousands of years of experience we understand that being human is not an easy task in any human culture. Being human is not an automated procedure by far. It seems that where being human is different from being animal takes place in the question on how we define and improve on our being human. Concepts as poverty and lack of civilization are often ascribed to being more like animals and wealth and civil behavior to the level of authority and control we take over our behavior and/or our biological functioning.

We call the process of being human 'organic' because the shapes of our lives are so multi-facetted and know so many possible alterations that lifestyles are often defined as a science, poetry or art. We also know that our lives are shaped by the boundaries of comfort, movability, environment, climate and so on.

Some cultures give people a more difficult time than others in defining themselves or in achievability of humanity. It often depends on how a culture defines being human. In modern forms of medicine it is accepted that the vision of being human defines how diseases are being understood, how strategies for cure can be developed and how health can be maintained or increased. It shows that we are primarily defined by culture and not just being bodies.

Modern globalist culture goes relatively easy on us. It allows us much stretch in our understandings. In fact it offers us so much stretch that our understanding often is diffuse, so that handling our health has increasing difficult problems to face.

Our being human in modern globalist culture is quite old fashioned and does not incorporate modern understanding about human beings. It is based on our body build mostly. It puts our chemistry first and our being human second. And although that is not wrong perse, it also isn't correct. It is not correct because it is not enough, not sufficient to deal with disease and health. It basically states that if we walk upright, have our head on the top, have two legs below and two arms on the side it is usually enough to qualify as human. Not being human and having this form is often named so because we behave monstrous or evil or uncompassionate. Having mental or physical handicaps is not seen as a reason to call someone un-human. Un-human if not inhuman immediately is associated with animal-like. Some redefine being human in different classes such as being civilized or hooligan; being upper class or working class; being educated or being un- educated. In this book we show you that being human can be fun but certainly involves the understanding that we are human 24-7.

Because this book mostly uses the differences and similarities between Chinese historical culture and global modern culture, of which China definitely is part, there will be many cultures we will not discuss. But the text is such constructed that it is easy to mirror your own culture in it if you do not recognize yourself in the content. By noting the difference with what is written in this text you understand there is a difference and you start describing it to yourself. As such the text contributes to your health due to increased cultural awareness. To do so is a good exercise in getting to know your culture better and thus to help you define how you and your kinsmen define health and disease yourself in the quest of improving your life situation. No cultural idea is by necessity wrong, but might need clarification before it can be properly contribute to your health. Where it goes wrong usually is due to lack of systematic understanding or a lack of being informed or because of stubborn insistence on personal opinions. These things in fact contribute too often to the formation of disease or decreased health. The fact that you have no pains or no tiredness does not have to mean you have no health related problems. Many problems manifest themselves in the experiental trends we go through. By the time we can define them as a disease usually we are already in an advanced stage of deterioration. When a disease comes acutely it can often be cured fast, but chronic diseases and complaints require long term management, study and physical practice to help develop clarity and reshape the tools of our body to live long and generate happiness. To be short: in health issues there are no easy solutions, and this is what this book deals with. Easy solutions offer ways out of pain and misery but do not solve problems, in fact they contribute to often to prolonged difficulties, and sometimes even increase them.

This book is based on three ideas:

1) *The idea that to understand yourself and your health you need to study your culture to understand the rules to define yourself and being human.*

2) *Developing health is a gradual process but so is disease*
3) *We all can develop health in a natural way if given enough time and effort*

It requires a cultural change to help us accept the idea that health and disease are things we have a lot of control over by means of what we do and how we do things. For many people the idea that we are responsible for what we achieve in health and disease is irreconcilable with the idea of for instance genetic disposition. But health is not only absence of disease, it is also in how we deal and incorporate disease in our daily life and society.

So, the experience that understanding your own culture is not as easy as it seems. Partly this is because your language and cultural habits define what you are allowed to know and not to know, and that is also about your culture. Knowledge, truth and so on are therefore narrowly defined by your culture and thus knowledge and truth are only relative values.

Studying a truly alien culture can help you to redefine your own culture and thus come to new and often revealing understandings. In my own study of Chinese culture I definitely started thinking a lot about my own culture, not in terms of vague criticism based on a certain un happiness, but on real valuable arguments that contributed to my wellbeing.

Summarizing: even if you disagree with the content or manners of your culture you do this according to preset understandings. For instance: modern biology knows the mind and the body are finely intertwined and cannot function without each other. But although it recognizes the thinking mind is part of human biology, the mind is still mostly treated as a guest to the body as defined by Christian religious doctrine that states that the self is part of the body of god and thus of a different nature then the body. Christianity defines the self as a thing independent from the reality around it. This thought originates in Ancient Greek thinking, such as from Plato. The Platonic thought is also the root of Buddhism, which is essential part of Chinese historical culture. Plato considered the mind as somewhat fuzzy and deluded and only able to understand indirect truths. In Buddhism knowing truth directly means you are enlightened and have overcome interdependent human existence. These are forms of individualism. Being human in the one is seen as being incapable of understanding reality, while in the other being human is being understood as enlightened or able to be enlightened. In all three visions we see that the self is seen as a thing (in Chinese the word for thing is dongxi, which means east-west, originally referring to the relationship we have with objects based on our feelings and ethics).

Things the west and the east agree upon are simple to define: human beings have bodies, and they can think. The nature of the mind and the methods the mind applies to think are not perceived as wholly similar. The west holds the idea that humans have a divine immortal soul that predates our being human. The east holds the idea that people have hun and po that check our actions and report the goodness of us at the moment of death to Heaven and Earth, during life every month they go report our badness. Chinese ancient culture had no idea of a soul as such. But it is believed by Buddhists and Daoists that through practice something of us can be produced or salvaged to continue in some form of existence after death. Science sees the body as a machine, the east believes the body is a reflection of nature of the self and nature at large. Christians believe the soul is innate goodness and the body is naturally bad. Confucianism states that people need education to become good or maintain goodness. Christianity and Islam say that people can only find peace in unity with god while the east is more unified on people finding peace when they follow the ordering of nature at large, and so on and so on. The list of differences is endless, while the list of similarities is only fractional of that. These differences have consequences that outwardly might look the same but inwardly are directed towards completely un-similar outcomes. Western biology is about the perfection or lack of perfection of the source of what makes us human, while Eastern ancient biology is about the ideal of what we can accomplish and actually achieve of it what makes us human. In the west because the body is seen as biological machine, technology is the natural tool to improve our body. In the ancient eastern view the body was noted as an expression of earth and its qi, and it is therefore through behavior that it can be molded to allow for the development of new possibilities and destinies.

In Chinese culture we see for that the self is not so much defined as a thing inhabiting the body, but as defined by its relationships (guanxi). The self is therefore more of a social event. The Chinese medicine/biology vision of the mind is seen as build from the level of water and qi up to the imaginations and thoughts and feelings that rule our daily life. It is therefore deeply rooted in being body. It sees emotive and physical functions as deeply entwined if not identical. It defines the physical structures therefore primarily in relationship to their contribution in being human or person. On top of that an ethical component (hunpo) that roots in heaven, earth and society checks our being human and determines our faith. Being human therefore is not only defined by being body, but also by his faith. All these factors are not necessarily fixed too. They can be altered, although change usually is not an easy process because it takes time and effort.

These definitions stand far away from how people experience themselves. Usually people in any culture experience themselves as rather random events. Their health and even the content of their feelings and thoughts seems outside their control. People can worry about that a lot, age early, can be plagued by small sufferings and large impacts of disease, or simply go crazy. This book is about that not being necessary. If we study culture we know the pathway to health because we make a science out of living. We construct ourselves according to this model or that. This book then does not give you rules about how to think or act, but gives you tools from which you can construct yourself and your health based on whatever culture you choose to take from.

Developing tools for self-experience and to alter the trends of health require to think as ourselves as some sort of system with very flexible parameters. So many details are not very much fixed. But in fact if we work in stages we can even develop super health even when starting from scratch. To a degree we can even predict which learning stage will take how much time. Building health is much like building a platform on which another platform can be build, and then another and so on, much like the pyramids in Middle America and China.

Constructing yourself is a life-long task, maintaining and developing your health is the same task. It happens if you like it or not. If you do not do anything you give in to randomness and chance and that is a self-constructing method in itself. It also allows insurance banks to earn billions at your expense, finance a medical industry and shapes political policy. You may not be aware of it but in most countries freedom stops where health stops. Cancelling human rights for freedom takes place on the level of health. Individual rights do usually not count when you are ruled by disease, or worse, become a hazard to your environment. Moreover, when diseased or suffering even from minor discomforts a generous portion of our abilities to do as we want and/or must is by nature taken away by ourselves. So there are good reasons to en masse exercise our right to be healthy as defined by the World Health Organization. Being healthy is a huge element of being and feeling free.

In any culture we see that some people do very good in making the most of their lives and many others do much less so. It seems to be much to depend on coincidence, luck and faith if life is going to be good to us or not. But if we try to look objectively at ourselves we see that indeed our lives often are quite accidental. The result of that is that we have too often surrender to the effect that circumstances have on us, such as a wrong quality meal in a restaurant, an autumn storm, stress at our job or in our relationships, or a pair of too narrow shoes. These all seem silly things to influence us, but they do.

This book wishes to hand you simple tools to improve your quality of life by means of small tools based on the practice and exercise of the functions of being us. By improving our sense organs, our understanding of our inner and outer body we can become more at ease with ourselves and less quick to be upset by our environment or emotions. More than that, we can fine-tune ourselves to the point where we become professional human beings, and function in accordance to our specs as given by our biological possibilities. This means being less often sick, aging more slowly and more gracefully and being generally more supportive to other human beings.

The observations and proposed skills in this books are based on scientific observations as well as on China's ancient Daoist immortality traditions and the naturalist biology underpinning Chinese medicine. These are a mixed biological/cultural/philosophical/medical science in themselves. In respect to the idealism about being human they match seamlessly although their visions on the body and being a person varies significantly.

Chinese pre-modern biology is by nature highly idealist, while western biology is constructed around a certain fatalist outlook on reality: it is often said that our destiny is in the genes or phenotypes. In Chinese biology it is suggested that people can be so much more by conditioning them (both Mencius and Xunzi agree on that part and they are not in disagreement with the huangdineijing suwen chapter 1 that says that people are confused and diseased due to circumstances that lead them to give in to feelings of anger, fear and desire). The huangdineijing is the oldest medicine textbook that follows a consistent cultural theory in its description of health and disease that is still in use. Translated it means something like: `the way how the internals are organized according to the the king of yellow/earth'. It is a compilation of medical visions from a wide geographic area that became united because of the way how yin yang theory, wuxing theory, sancao theory and some ten other significant theories were put in conjunction to each other as a result of certain breakthroughs in logic about 2500 years ago. This period we can see as the beginning of Chinese historical culture. Like the west ofcourse it has a history that goes back tens of thousands of years and crosses the boundaries of modern humans to pre-modern humans such as Neandertals and Cro-magnons, but these do not count as argument. It is this time that defines our understanding of Chinese culture. Before that time there was simply another cultural group which we call preconditions for the formation of Chinese culture. In the same ways Egyptian and Assyrian cultures are not western cultures because in the Greek classical times the formation of western culture took place out of these other ones.

Later cultural change in either cultures did not significant alter the content, but the content was different from before. Chinese culture defined itself by means of its examples and its ideals. Theory therefore expresses an ideal and reality is to aim to fulfill that ideal. Health development then is in achieving ideal health, which is called 'returning to the origin'. Returning to the origin does not mean going back to the beginning. It means going to realize what is ideal; a-priori.

Greek culture defined that the world is built from atoms, called earth water, fire and air. Where Chinese culture follows ideas, western culture describes even ideas on the basis of their thing- ness. We still construct our theories according to the method of building blocks. In western biology we are seen as conditioned by genes, circumstances etc, these are constructed from elements that add up to each other. Our sentences and words as constructed from letters follow that same logic of thing-ness. Because outcomes are supposed to be as fundamental as their causes we look for universals. The way to do so is by means of average values, so we are measured by statistical presence. So our averageness is seen as standard, not the thing as it is or can be. Habits are therefore the measure of truth in statistics. It is not always easy to accept the difference and also face the consequences of the one belief or the other. In fact if the first belief looks more attractive, this is a good time to live because nowadays we can grow into alien cultures as a lifestyle choice.

That was something our ancestors generally did not have as an option. It offers us new tools to deal with our discomforts when we learn to deal with these cultural tools under discipline. Using such tools for a few weeks does not make them useful. All health tools are lifestyle tools.

Every science is by nature imperfect and riddled with flaws. It is why searching for truth is so important in many cultures. Ofcourse it is also the flaw of western science. You can upset scientists very much by being very different from others in your functioning. One time in a hospital I took a breathing test.

The physician couldn't hear my breathing after he ordered me 4x that I should breathe. I was breathing but I needed two minutes for one breath. He expected to hear rattling noises and so on from the stressful breathing people normally have with 15-25 breaths a minute. But in Chinese biology that is seen as a sign of stress. A healthy breath goes slow and soundless.

That breath also goes together with a smooth plain mood. To be different at something than the average is therefore at times explained as a disease factor and not necessarily as a possible function of being human. Many of our diseases are unchecked talents that got out of hand because of not understanding them properly and not exercising them properly.

This is also the reason why I set out to write the book in your hand when I got invited to write one book for English and Chinese language audiences. If I can help this way that people come to recognize their possibilities and set out to improve themselves a bit, the general quality of life on the whole planet can be changed. To achieve this change is your personal Daoland program. After all, you are the master and source of your life.

Daoland self-programming

The purpose of your Daoland program is to help you build defense against disease, tear and wear, stress, inattentiveness at life's crucial moments and your own darker sides in an organic and natural way. It also intent's to fine-tune and improve capacities you already seem to have by nature so that you can rely on them more. Thirdly, the program will introduce skills and perspectives you didn't know about yet, and for you personally it can be quite innovative.

In life, it is not enough to have talents, we all have them. Talent can be defined as a natural ability to do something. Suzanne van de Groep wrote at LeidenUniversityblog.nl in 2018 that "we all know someone who has a natural gift of this kind: that person who can draw the most beautiful portraits or has an exceptional singing voice. To some, this definition of talent may sound frighteningly deterministic: can you only be successful if you have a natural gift for something?" What se wrote aboiut in that blog is that just talent will not help you much. I have friends that have talents, but their life still didn't beome a great success. I am not saying they aren't happy, but they could have done more with their life to support their fellow beings, and indirectly themselves too. Talent isn't a bragging factor. It is a potential, a potential energy, to mention a term from physics. In modern spirituality and pop esoterics people often speak of energy they can feel. You might be one of them. But energy is the talent that you can feel but cannot bring to fruition. A talent needs to be cultivated through learning. This book shows you to hone the talent to be healthy. These are the other factors that contribute to success:

- *Effort*: the degree of activity you invest to achieve your goals. You could even say that without effort, your talents are wasted: they will not develop further or help you to achieve your goals. To be successful,
- *Ambition*: it is also important to realize what your goals are and to really want to achieve them (i.e., to be ambitious). So, even though talents may be very important to succeed,
- Morality: the choises we make on how we develop our talents and what we use them for is a counterpoint in the willingness to hone your talent. Not using your talent can be a loss for the community and yourself.

I think you will agree that it is only when combined with effort and ambition that your talents will really blossom, leading to success.

It is important to use and hone our talents into professional skills to have happier and more successful lives. Health in this definition is just a professional skill.

Successful lives contribute to the welfare of all living beings, not only our own of those in our circle of friends or family. Our biology shows that we all have many potential talents available in a trove that Daoists call 'our original nature'. By taxing and training these talents our lives will be more full, active and happy. We also discover that there are many talents to be discovered waiting for us beyond the horizon of what we now feel possible for us. When well informed we can keep developing us in any direction we require development. Human beings are very versatile and flexible in our adaptions. It is our scavenger heritage. We are creatures that can flourish when we are forced to live economically. We enjoy finding ways to deal with problems or solve problems. We enjoy that as a team and by ourselves.

This text introduces ideas and reflections upon Chinese medicine and yangsheng ideas, drawing also on Western and Chinese spiritual ideas, traditions and practices; emphasizing the differences and highlighting the benefits of these differences to help all humans forward in being human. You have to remember that no cultural science is better than another. All cultures are born from trial and error and error is just as common as success and some errors are just simply funny in how they are continuously recreated in clinic, such as antibiotics, cupping and scraping techniques. It doesn't take away that in rare cases they are useful, but they are in themselves a bad idea, however commonly used. What we now do is take a look at all the ideas and look for what we can do and how they can be explained. It does not mean it is the only explanation. Sharing each others experiences is important this process. You will see that every cultural input when consistently used will give different outcomes, and that is a key element of Daoland learning: to validate the concept of culture in formation of knowledge and science.

Knowledge comes to us in different layers:

- *Universal knowledge (humans are alive, at nights some lights are present in a dark background)*
- *Cultural layer of common knowledge (regionally or ethnically determined)*
- *Personal knowledge (experience)*

Each of these layers has its own value. Cultural layers dress up universal knowledge but also give direction to that knowledge. That directionality is what makes knowledge into a science because it lets us ask questions. The question about quantum elements in space is therefore not universal because the question comes forth from the question what is god and what is god not, which is typical European. Indian culture never asked the same question, although with some creativity we could imagine it to be part of ancient classics. But even then it remains cultural science, not universal. You have to also realize that animals reason from universal knowledge. Culturally or personally they add very little to the knowledge they carry with them all their life.

Introduction to causes

This book is about living a natural lifestyle as part of becoming healthy. In effect we have two choices in regard to health:

artificially induced health and naturally induced. Ofcourse you have to make a consistent choice in this to not confuse your system. Confusion creates conflict and conflict generates ailment.

I therefore invite you to ask questions about what is natural, what is a lifestyle, and what is the general use of lifestyles? Before you read any further, write your ideas about this on an A4 so that you have unalterable proof of what you think about that right now. Classify your knowledge under universal, cultural or personal.

It is somewhat fashionable to live a natural lifestyle. We have to remember that a natural lifestyle uses elements of nature but is not how we would live when living in nature. Life in nature often is harsh, demanding and often full of poverty or hunger. People living in nature are often not environmentally aware, in contrast to what we think, but they pollute nature less because they have no industrial production of things, crèmes and so on. The beauty and intensity of cultural expressions (this is folklore) often tempts us to romanticize nature and read things into it that are not really there.

The romantic engagement with nature in fact is a sign of highly innovative technological and scientific thinking, weather we look at the Chinese or Japanese gardens or the European spa resorts. Health-wise the idea of 'natural' also is as much a criticism on nature as well as a romanticizing it. In fact 'natural' means we try to rely on possibilities nature offers us without nature itself maybe using these too. Natural means here: 'to do something by choice'. Natural here can then also be stretched in meaning, to involve being conscious on what one does and how one does it. Natural also means setting rules and regulations that border what we find acceptable or not. Natural therefore also regulates freedoms of choice we have and both opens areas of choice up as well that it closes others. The foregoing is why we talk about having a natural life-style that is in itself artificial but emulates natural objects/processes. It usually is not a lifestyle that is the same as from people who have no choice but to deal with nature as part of survival.

Both in East and west there are questions about how to live a natural lifestyle and so far few realize that living a natural lifestyle is living up to your natural potential, not necessarily living leisurely, which is often the image of the person who has achieved mastership in being human in the east. In the west many interpret living naturally as living on impulses. But in fact both lifestyles leave us vulnerable to influences that daily come upon us from the environment, multi-media and society at large. The principle of natural then is not so simple as the word natural seems to suggest. 'Natural' in western conception means in accordance with nature or natural law or as how we can see it happening in nature as well. In Chinese language 'Ziran' follows the principle of 'being as it should be by itself', which implies fitting in the larger string of things and events, and thus contributing to the grandness of existence at large. In the west Natural follows laws of cause and effect, and in Chinese history Ziran indicated being free of interdependent origination and virtuously following the Dao of heaven and earth.

Lifestyle is a much more easy concept to explain. A lifestyle is the method someone uses to find completion in one's life. It is in modern life the right of each person to design his or her own lifestyle in relationship to the goals of global society at large, and hopefully to the benefit of all involved.

The book offers some insights in that field from east and west. It does not proscribe rules about what to do, but it invites you to investigate what you could do and make work for you and your environment and thus to design for yourself a healthy lifestyle. Although the basis of its ideas and methods originate in China I am myself not originally Chinese. I can call myself culturally mixed, and as such I am part of a new world that we slowly see coming about around us. The book is therefore also a comment on ancient Chinese and Western/Modern/Chinese culture, a footnote that hopefully is of use to you.

East and west mutually influence each other

Usually we recognize that Chinese culture and European culture are two separated cultures. And that is in fact true. As a result of their relative separation they have developed different systems of viewing, judging and manipulating the world. The separation between the two cultures is not strict. Usually in the area between two cultures mixed and partial knowledge systems find ways to exist and compete, but usually connect to a preferred system. For instance Tibetan culture's preferred cultural knowledge system is Chinese, while Afghanistan's knowledge system already is much clearer European. Interchange has been larger the last few centuries, where it is considered that the west has had a dominant influence on China due to colonial processes taking place.

Ironically China has in the last few hundred years influenced the west in many ways as much as the west has influenced China. Improvements in chemistry, printing, agriculture, architecture, computing, mapmaking etc were possible due to interchange with China. But in spite of that being so, many meaningful things on both sides still remain elusive. This is where culture as determinants for knowledge comes most to the foreground.

In English language we struggle for instance with the difference and similarity between concepts such as energy and qi which are similar in some respects but very different in many other aspects even though their presence seem to be noticed in similar incidents. But because of their cultural difference therefore cannot naturally be that easily used to replace each other in translation.

To explain a bit on this: Qi is what we share with our environment but which we are ultimately ourselves responsible for to produce. Qi therefore is a result of something, of work being done, but inherent to a process too. Energy as a concept is a complicated mix between the idea that we have in us a 'breath of life' that is a gift of God and notions about electricity in physics. There is a similar case to be made for concepts such as 'shen and spirit' or 'xue and blood'. Shen is more like the hunter/prey's awareness, while spirit is the intent of the divine. Xue is a steppingstone in the process of developing earthlike yin as a root to produce yang that flows red in our vessels and marrow, while blood is a transport for nourishment, messages and poison that also happens to be red.

In a far future both culture's ideas will most likely have merged so much that seeing a difference will take specialists. The reason for this is the deep rooted desire from people to learn about the exotic, assimilate it and make it our own. Too often we step over the things we do not fully grasp and more often than not we eventually forget about them. That is often a pity because that way a lot gets lost in translation. The Daoland program allows to modify experiences depending on what cultural lifestyle you choose to live.

Modern Global Migration

Western Colonialism has shaken up world history and created a wave of migrations that at the point still is not reaching its end. It is not humanities first mass migration and it will most likely not be its last. But this one will have a huge impact on future science and culture. Your way of managing your health can benefit from that, as is the purpose of this program to help you with.

The current global migration creates curiosity and fear for the unknown but has also enriched societies all over the globe. We learned from it that people are driven by attachment to safety and experimentation with the unknown. Each person requires different dosage from each to feel comfortable.

At the same time global migration also drove some societies into extinction. No culture remained untouched by this event and it cannot be stopped or turned back too. It also allows us to re- envision our pasts and our futures. It allows us to reshape the products of the past and improve on it due to what we learn from other cultures. Daoland skills for instance are taken from a few thousand years of Chinese culture and made into an open source system which allows for multilevel interpretation and thus to investigate other culture's values and health systems. It means that the event allows us to have a fresh look at what we have created in the past, stand at the shoulders of our masters and aim to master ourselves too in a way that respects the masters the best way possible, namely by being better than them, not isolated as in the past, but as a joint force of helpful people working together at a better life on this little planet.

Modernization

Modernization -ofcourse- is a process long time in the making. But not even 50 years ago it was a process mostly instigated by governments and academies. That has changed since the internet has made the world a neighborhood, and you are part of that change if you like it or not.

Nowadays innovation is a private affair that academies are forced to follow and governments regulate after things occurred and show uncontrollable growth. Some examples are the internet, the quickly developing new-age healthcare market, the drugs and medicines market, and commercial spaceflight. As part of the Daoland program we organize our own academic level education next to general supportive healthcare programs accessible for everyone and directly showing results in self-generated improvements. 50 years ago that was simply impossible, but now it is not only possible, but similar initiatives take place all over the globe. It thrives on exotism and revivalism as well as on the need to be modern and up to date with the events of the world so that we do not loose out on its new benefits. These two are powerful shapers of culture and science. we can shortlist them also as curiosity and conservatism.

Exotism and revivalism

In China exoticism did lead to partial abandonment of the past and as a result also revivalist movements. Revivalist movements have one big problem, they look at the past from a revised perspective while claiming to know the past. I once had an argument with a Chinese hospital director who claimed I could not understand Chinese culture because I am not Chinese. As a counter argument I brought up that neither was he. He cited the Huangdineijing and other classics to show his knowledge. But being part of a tradition is more in its skills then in its knowledge of classics recitation. Modern practice in Chinese medicine classics is deeply influenced by western biology and hospital management. Diagnosis, anatomy, tools, environment, everything has become westernized. So have his clothing, his housing conditions, his watch, wallet, money and so on. So in all respects he is a westerner like me. He just doesn't feel a westerner. Because of long standing resentment and an education system that not only teaches people to be part of their culture but also keeps pointing to enemies of that culture difference between East Asians and Westerners is deeply felt, even though in all practical life they have become deeply western in most aspects of life and possibilities in life choices. In fact, trying to revive ancient practices is in China often frowned upon. It is discussed as being useful, but all is tested through 'scientific reasoning' which is a censorship system based on western modes of thought. Actual people still living in the past are studied as part of folklore. It is also the same as happens in the west. Worse, the censorship is also used to romanticize Chinese history by these same revivalists. What they tell themselves and their audiences all over the world is not necessarily wrong but it is certainly not right. Let us go through a few examples:

Modern Chinese medicine makes the claim of being 5000 years old, but that is a fabrication based on easily engaged misunderstandings. Chinese medicine as it is practiced today is a typical 20th century phenomenon and thus it is new. But it has a developmental history that stretches back maybe 10.000 years. But because the idea of China was only created in the warring states period, Chinese medicine as such is only about 2500 years old. It is Chinese because of the use of combined basic theories such as wuxing, yinyang, sancao etc. (Altogether there are 13 such theories which not all are used in modern Chinese medicine clinic. In the revial of Chinese medicine they discuss only two or three, and then mostly in the context of western chemistry and Hegelian dialectics. They are discussed in the Daoland online university courses). So in fact there are three distinct Chinese medicines that are not at all on a parr:

Period	*typical*
Pre-Chinese medicine	Based on witchcraft, combining spells and potions without a defining theory, although some ideas were rudimentary present in its later periods
Chinese medicine	Based on concepts as qi, yinyang, wuxing, heaven-earth-man, Confucianism, Daoism and Buddhism etc. Defined by health theory
New China Chinese medicine	Redefined scientific Chinese medicine, testable according to non- Chinese anatomy and physiology, disease theory, chemistry and physics. Defined by disease theory

Modern Chinese ancient Medicine in many ways is a revised medicine that follows many western scientific lines of reasoning as a guided attempt to modernize Chinese Medicine and keep up with exotic findings by western science. These changes go so far that some call it a western medicine with Chinese features. Likewise in traditional Chinese sports: Currently many gongfu (such as wushu and taijiquan) teachers use terminology from western ballet and physiotherapy to explain their practice. For instance the method of hanging yourself on a thread from baihui. Baihui means '100 returnings'. It is indicative for the way how Chinese culture thinks about the body. It says that if the head is placed properly then we feel like coming home to ourselves. Baihui is an acupuncture point on the midline of the skull. Baihui's location is precisely described. The crown -which is a western concept- is much vaguer in description of location. It also has no other function then being the top of the body, or has it? It is part of the sink line going down the trunk from the point in question to Huiyin, Huiyin is located at where biology locates the perineum, between the sexual organs and anus. It is the focus of the lower diaphragm that holds our interior body in place. Hui yin means 'collection of yins, which means the water of the body and the mass/substance of the body. As such it is in function opposite from huiyin and they both deal with water and stuff.

It is in ballet the method to allow the dancer to connect with God and be a puppet of God by hanging on a string from the crown. In fact that is why it is called the crown. It creates the typical swan like floating movements as if flying. It metaphysically makes people into marionettes that are being guided by Gods hand. It is also commonly used as a result of that to correct people on bad posture. The method is defended as scientific in for instance physio-therapeutics. It belongs to the category of accepted cultural knowledge. Therefore in east and west many modern Gongfu people use physiotherapeutic theory without knowing. And not only in how to correct posture.

Their explanation of Li-muscle power, Yi-intent and Qi (we come to that later) often is skewed unintentionally by modernization when they follow this description. In original Chinese cultural context the had was to be propped up so that baihui would be turned to heaven and function in the way a vase has an opening to poor water in. in people the baihui, not the crown is where heaven can be let in to the body so that we can collect it and interpret the will of heaven. I hope the reader understand that the difference is more than just semantics. It also allows the body to hold the musculature in different ways, but it also generates a different feel of the whole of the body. In the 'ballet-way' emotive perception is more easy to develop. While in the 'martial-way' a more capacity perception is more easy to develop. The directionality of muscular use also is different. In the one the bones are central and the muscles hang on the bones. In the other the muscles are central and the bones hang inside the muscles.

The truth is that modernization doesn't necessarily mean becoming better or worse. It means things change. It also means some essential insights in the human condition run the risk of becoming lost. Current Chinese martial arts and medicine perception, practice and theories hoovers between western and original theories. Recent recognition of Chinese medicine as world heritage has only made that more clear. As such we see that there is a modern China and a historical \ China and they are not necessarily believing the same things, even if they use the same words. Being Chinese many of these changes do not need to be recognized. Likewise as a westerner you do not know the intricacies from Chinese cultural views and uses, so you have to make do with what Chinese people recognize in your culture to explain themselves... we see the difficulty here...? What is interesting though is what takes place on the fringe between the boundaries we just outlined. This book is written on these boundaries and can therefore show how much ideas integrate, separate and cause renewal in cultural views, medicine and sports on both sides of the cultural separation. What we see is that development of our understanding is closely interlinked with the development of modern personal health management skills.

In western countries Chinese medicine and Martial arts have become very popular indeed, be they small in importance. Because western law only partially recognizes the rights of Chinese medicine practice practitioners have been struggling for their professional survival often leaning heavily on western laboratory research to prove its validity. What I said above about the Chinese situation therefore doubly so is relevant for the western situation. As a result many Chinese medicine concepts are explained out of context, leading to strange paradoxes when you try to understand the medicine science. Wushu and taijiquan as part of that suffers even a harder lot because the west doesn't place martial arts in a cultural moral context as China does even though teachers refer to that part. Although the west shows research that practice of martial arts is good for health or can increase learning ability and health status, wushu is generally seen as something suitable for the lower classes of society and children, and not really the art form which it can be too. The reason why people wish to learn about these things in fact is the typically Chinese-ness of it and not its western contribution, which often is not recognized or explained. So its organizational needs and the curiosity that cause people to want to know about it are not of the same kind.

What is most important is that everybody focuses on competitive sports and clinical medicine application, while in fact Chinese biology and health practice are the core of what is Chinese in Chinese medicine and sports. It becomes Chinese sports because of the division in Neigong (inward practice) and Waigong (outward practice), which each have their own learning program which is not in the movements but in the embodiment of principles. Neigong and waigong division also runs through Chinese medicine. Herbal medicine is waidan (externally made medicine), but through internal practice (neidan, internally made medicine) its efficiency can be made to improve significantly. Neidan is nothing else then self-regulation of normal body functions which require attention, outward movement and inward movement in close coordination.

From this it is obvious that gongfu has many aspects that are too important to not incorporate in any sports or health program. To summarize, below we see a short summary of the benefits of a balanced gongfu program. The cool thing about Daoland healthcare is that it even manages to incorporate these aspects in a simple thing like a massage, or an acupuncture facelift.

Major Functions of Chinese martial arts	**Particulars**
Self-defense/offense	Applications to deal with attackers to discourage or disable
Fitness practice	Endurance and stamina development under stress by pressure, speed, balance based challenges
Postural development	Maximizing postural space and radiance
Personality development	Ethical behavior, courage, self-confidence
Intellectual development	Strategic planning, predictive capabilities, mechanical insight, discernment, creative development and sense of aesthetics and appropriateness
Health and balance	Well-being, spatial understanding, directional understanding, sense of symmetry and a-symmetry, grasp of own body form and ability
Neigong	Internal process and experiential development, root-process of life development

Western sports or medicine does not have that. They have feedback and feedforward techniques based on mechanical measurement. Self-observation in neigong and waigong is the same. We have all the measurement equipment already build into ourselves in the form of our sense organs and awareness, so we can save money on not having to buy it. We just need to learn to read the signs. But that doesn't take much time, we already have some skills, and the more healthy we become the better developed our skills will be. Where a normal person sees one thing, a healthy person sees two or more.

Sports and medicine in Chinese medicine are never divided. Likewise for beauty treatment. The idea that health is the root of beauty is deeply engrained in Chinese beauty techniques, so Chinese beauty techniques are not just cosmetic, but aim to help restore health as well. Chinese medicine and health techniques are based on understanding of the relationships between substance and movement.

Some say that westerners cannot understand Chinese culture or vice versa that Chinese people are likely to misjudge western culture. But the truth is that individual understanding is not that relevant. Understanding is something negotiated between all of us. It is in our language, habits and behavior. We all struggle to come to grips with our lives, our culture and our science. Life is quite short and so full of experiences that we often forget that we as a species create understanding, and not as individuals, so that our actions should in general take each others difficulties in account. The struggle with meaning is relevant only if it provides a better living environment, peace and health for everyone. I feel therefore very happy that I am allowed to explain a few thoughts of myself and from the people who serve as my peers, my examples or teachers. I am happily obliged to share with you the resulting applications which we summarize under the Daoland health care system. Daoland contains an extensive self-learning experience by means of sports and care programs.

Yangsheng in a global perspective

This modern world is a new reality where we can freely choose cultural models to learn from. It is a new form of emancipation, that of equality of culture. So far that is not the case. There is only one scientific model acceptable for instance, that is following strict Christian paradigms of an ontological universe, that is, a universe that originates from the same point where time started. The Chinese model follows a more diffuse origin model. The origin takes place all the time. The paradigms of a culture are a scientific culmination of observations about the nature of things.

Because cultures are born out of different circumstances they see things different. Even though we have the same bodies, there are difference in detail and principle in about everything. These differences are important, because they teach us about the human condition. Take health for instance. Pre-modern Chinese and modern western concepts of health are by no means comparable. Even the visions about anatomy and physiology are different so although we look similar we have different bodies based on our cultural views and the therefrom originating experiences of ourselves. What is interesting is that one culture's health might be another culture's abnormality. Realizing this means we are learning about health in relationship to being human.

Health is not an absolute. Health is a relative. Health relates to understanding, so does disease in many cases. In western view for instance health and disease are two separate entities. But in the Chinese view disease and health often are two different continua. In measurements you might be ill but in actual practice you are healthy. I give you an example of a Dutch student I once had. She suffered cramps in her limbs and felt often wooly under her feet. I let her do particular not too easy exercises and meditations and her condition greatly improved to the point where the symptoms almost disappeared. She was a confident and promising student. Then she went on holiday and forgot to practice. Symptoms recurred and she went to a physician, who made the diagnosis she has multiple sclerosis, which is incurable. She was angry with me for not having told her that she had this terrible disease, she quitted practice and she never recovered. What she suffered was being part of a knowledge system. The knowledge system we have condemns everything that does not fit in it. What we usually therefore say about other cultures is a criticism, and not an understanding. What I mean to say is that language, disease theory etc is a judgment system. It makes us believe things. Not telling her made her experience herself as healthy. If she would have kept up practice she maybe would have aged happily until a point where it was not so relevant anymore that she had an incurable disease. Maybe she would actually have cured herself. It is for this reason and others why Daoland focus is on restoring health and not on curing disease, just like Chinese medicine from the past used to do.

Chinese medicine traditionally revolves around the idea that people require continuous involvement in health practice to acquire and develop health. When diseased people are found to be in a certain level of confusion that then counts as the main reason why it is difficult to restore health. The confusion works as a distractor, or obstruction of the curative process. Especially for chronic diseases being sick is a habit of the body, and/or the person, and because habits are difficult to change/brake, it requires disciplinary actions to do so. The more passive a person is in the process the less likely a cure will occur, although an improvement is possible. A cure would mean no recurrence of the problem, no side effects or derivate of the problem causing new syndromes. Improvement or even hiding of the original complaint or absence of for instance pain does not equal cure. It could as well mean that medication has clouded your mind so much you do not notice the original complain anymore that much, as is for instance the case with painkillers, anti-depressants or anti-convulsives.

Of this confusion traditionally business-people eagerly make use to earn some cash by calling themselves doctors or masters of ancient secrets. They do this by means of confirming the confusion and promising cures for which our effort is minimal. Usually that is done in the form of giving medication. Medication can help a curative process, but cannot achieve cure by itself. The same with many other medicinal techniques, they can help you underway but cannot solve your problems, according to Chinese medicine theory. Skills like taiji, meditation, yoga, gongfu, qigong, breathing exercises and so on likewise can only get you so far, but they are the primary tools for you to develop the internal skills that are required to develop and maintain good health. If the practices help depends a lot on the kind of instructions you get. In modern yoga it is often advised to breathe through a tension, that originates in autogenic training. In Chinese medicine we are advised against that due to the long-term consequences of giving too much specific attention to a traumatized spot inside ourselves. It is said you this way feed it and make it stronger and more likely to return. The direct approach to healing is not always the most useful. Often the indirect approach is more effective to deal with problems. In qigong we teach people that whatever location you concentrate on things start accumulate. Accumulation eventually leads to obstruction and stagnation or even infection or smoldering heat. Only a few places allow to accumulate without stagnation. Concentration on places should normally go shallowly as not to cause problems. When one's focus is on problems one likely reinforces the roots of that problem and makes it harder to cure. Western style is on looking for details to correct the chain of things. Chinese style is in generalizing to let the details get guided by the needs of the whole.

Every new practice reinvents history, that is, the reality of things. We just try to connect to originally intended meanings: In doing so we also create new science, new policies and dreams. Daoland science is both about western and Chinese science, but can be open to all other cultural meanings too. As a westerner I do see these meanings in a slightly different light then many of my Chinese counterparts. Because of my deep involvement with Chinese people I also see these meanings in a slightly different light then most of my western counterparts. I hope it brings you many benefits

There is only one study

If we are fair about our lives we see that only one thing really matters, and that is life. Being successful, rich, having a big house or car, spouse etc is all not that important, even though we may enjoy its presence greatly. People construct their natures and behaviors to the extent of corruption and purity just to get a bit more of life. To maintain life we eat, drink, breathe and move around, just like bugs and algae's do. We have specialized appendages and sense organs to do this in the particular way only humans do.

The next thing that matters to people is not feeling alone, and thus to feel connected. From the way how we live together in groups from the beginning we clearly feel better in numbers and it is therefore no surprise that we developed mathematics and other number arts from the beginning of the rise of our intelligence. In a group we also feel more like learning, we feel competitive and take the lead of our lives in many different ways. We even go so far as developing harmful behavior if it brings us up into a group as a leader in one way or another. In that sense, there are as many forms of leadership as there are people. To be real about the situations we live in: we are all king of our own kingdom. We might feel powerless in the way how our life is going, but that feeling is one way to confirm what I just tell you here: life is a constructed experience. We cannot change it rapidly, but over time we can build tools to greatly improve on our lives. If we are conscious of it or not, in general terms we can state that we are always in control, even if it is only in giving our control to people or things that harm us. That is why we are all kings in our own country. How we rule that country is up to us. In Daoism they use the adagium: the reality outside ourselves we find reflected in the experience of the reality inside ourselves.

Our experiences and conceptions are highly malleable. We are gullible enough to believe anything, so we can also come to believe truly helpful things if we want too. All you need is to develop tools to investigate things and come to questions the things you think you already know. Mostly you find you only know fragments of ideas. This partial understanding of things is unsystematic, confusing and disease and discomfort creating. It gives us the feeling of being out of control. It does not allow us to develop a way out other the through dependency. Daoland aims to let you know yourself through independency: be a sovereign king in your own country, not a puppet-king.

When are we puppet-kings? As a people we are alternating selfish, altruist and destructive however it seems suitable to the options we recognize in our life to connect with people. Even when we get isolated, our resulting depressions are signs of feeling connected, although we do not feel it is an appropriate form of connectedness. Even when we get hospitalized we feel connected because our disease connects us with a huge staff that serves us. It hardly ever happens that someone gets disconnected from being human, although we blame ourselves and others often from being exactly that. To get out of that misconception we follow Laozi, who said 2500 years ago that Dao is always close to us so we are never truly lost. Developing health can start with practicing something small but beneficial. Gradually it gains power and dilutes our bad habits.

The third thing that matters to us is creating hierarchy in our lives. Although we feel close to the whole of our community, culture, humanity or nature, we seem to have a need to make some elements more important than others. We call this understanding of hierarchy the natural order of things. Some things seem to precede other things and some things we attach more deeply to then others. Some attach to the relationship we hold with things or people and other attach more to the things or people themselves. This division is at least as important to us as the gender difference. If we are male of female determines a lot of how we feel about things. For instance being a man makes you less sensitive on the emotional level because it is not useful for a man to cry while killing rabbits for food. Although some people try to be non-hierarchical, that attempt in itself creates a hierarchy. Mozi is a famous Chinese example in his suggestion that we should love everyone equal. Some modern political and social movements active in the world try to achieve the same. For instance: Democracy and Communism strife in their ideologies for the same goal of non-hierarchical equality. When we are healthy we generally feel quite comfortable about anything and that is probably the most non-hierarchical we ever get.

So what we can conclude from the above? Indeed, although we have created many educational institutions that teach us all kinds of facts and skills which all are very useful, there is only one study: the study of life. All other studies flow out of that study and are only useful to us if they support the study and practice of life.

The purpose of life is only to keep on living. There is not much to it. It is inherent to existence. A rock doesn't just like that stop existing. The rock maybe is not aware of its existence but exists nevertheless. We as conscious beings can see ourselves progress rather fast through the stages of beginning, maintenance and ending of our existence and the speed naturally worries us. If we allow ourselves to be a bit too passive in our life we feel our life is slipping away from us. We seem never ready enough.

Current trends in global warming, natural disasters, wars and other events only contribute to that feeling. Modern technology has all brought it to our doorsteps so that we as individuals can become witness of how existence affects us. We now can all clearly see that we never exist on our own. Buddhism and Daoism each expounded on theories of interdependent origination. Modern physics likewise shows a network of events to be the tapestry from which our existence and even our consciousness are constructed. If current global events show us anything, it is that we are easy to be influenced and affected by events on every level of existence. Most people came to understand that we have to make an effort to keep ourselves together, both as individuals as well as coherent helpful social communities. If we don't, either or both of them might fall apart. Our aging process itself is a proof of the reality of that process taking place. Observe how our old people age: are they a person or are they falling apart? When they fall apart, they have not been prepared for the aging. That is a social issue and a personal issue that we are all responsible for. Although we exist, we are no rocks.

To survive or to flourish

Above I said that the purpose of life is to keep on living. We see in nature that that life holds on to its precious existence with a stubbornness which is both to be pitied and admired. We are part of that existence. The life of a anaerobic lifeform is no less significant then our own. It fights to survive as we do with the tools it has. Because we are constructed by the cooperation between many small beings we have developed many tools, but that means that for each person's actions many smaller life-forms depend on the correctness of these actions to survive or perish. If we do not take good care of ourselves they have not a good deal from living within us, but for them there is no other way out than to disease and die. That means we live not as persons but as codependent societies of beings.

Throughout history much of people's lives were much of the same. It was not that we were poor, but for many there were not enough resources to create long and healthy lives. The happiness of the poor is often romanticized, but it ius usually the rich who do that, and not the poor. Economy nowadays seems very important to help us sustain a comfortable life in a large city, but for most of our history economy was about fair share and exchange in small communities depending on the local circumstances of climate, earth fertility and occurrence of disasters.

It is not that the knowledge was not available on how to live healthy, often it was. But history teaches us that health was often associated with the supernatural because it was so rare a quality to acquire. As a result nobody really knew what powers a healthy person could have over the unhealthy and malnutritioned.

The Chinese culture by means of the Huangdineijing associated good health with everlasting life. European and Arabic areas too associated immortality as of the healthy. In the first culture immortality was the result of paying attention to the environment and avoiding distractions that would lead one away from being harmonious part of it. In the second immortal health was the result of being united with God. In the Islamic/ Christian culture mystical rapture was therefore sometimes of a larger importance as proof of health, while in the east an aloof detachment was seen as a good chance that health could be acquired. In modern cities we see that in private time often rapture is being sought by means of intoxication. Rapture is the result of overheating our system, speeding ourselves up so to say. New Age people often speak of living on higher frequencies. The disadvantage is that we destabilize our emotions and create more vulnerability to suggestion, even though whatever we feel feels more as truth. The Chinese ancient system is based on a gradual increase of inward pressure which allows us to develop a continuous clarity which is a high in its own way, but then comparable to the high of lying on your back floating in lukewarm water and enjoying the sun. it is the kind of fun babies are supposed to have when in their mother's womb.

What we need and what we feel we need

Being part of a European society I was raised with wealth around me as history had never known before in a family that did economically not even rank that well. We were relatively spoken not very rich at home, but we were collecting things.

In this modern time more and more nations gradually create wealth out of their endless human resources. Thus, more and more people are able to live a life like I myself had or even better. It also means they will have more time spent in being educated and learning about the world, other cultures, alternative lifestyles. Many of these people will learn the same as I did, namely that there is more to life than just surviving.

Surviving as a principle is based on struggle. It means that the parameters of survival are so tight that there is no time for anything else than assuring existence. In a way we might say that relative abundance of resources makes life for a species more easy. When life is easy cultures can come about in a species, such as the building habits of some species of birds, or the eating habits of chimpanzees. It requires much time to actually come to an argument about things where the discussion is not a mere bullying or blackmailing of the other to be right. The discovery of reasonability is probably one of the most important ones of our long shared history. It is more important than language because it requires cooperation and mutual understanding to be reasonable. But when we started writing we started to create artificial memory to not forget what we were reasonable about. Now because of our relative wealth we can all be a bit more reasonable because we can be more safe in not having to survive every day.

Healthy and unhealthy conditions

In life there are moments of comfort and discomfort. It is important to realize these are all part of a healthy existence. If we are in good control of our health the moments of discomfort of any nature, be they of the body or of the feelings, will only be short lived. In health we feel comfortable, have no complicating feelings or thoughts and feel generally happy but not excessively so. We sleep easily and get out of bed smoothly; we do not usually get tired too much, even if we put a lot of effort in our activities. Our shen-awareness is clear and we can anticipate on possible health risks in tune with circumstances. Our body jing-construction is always vigilant and never sagging or tensing and our internal as well as our behavioral qi's are clear and purposeful. As a result our yuanjing (potential) is optimal. In case you read about Chinese medicine and sports before you see I explain Jing, Qi and Shen here as actions, as things happening and being done. I do not describe them as substances, but as something that develops substance in a way western culture would call second nature, something learned, acquired and inseparable from ourselves. I put guanxi (relations) in the center and not dongxi (things). Guanxi makes things into a system. Dongxi can be grouped.

It is important that I state these things for the progress of this book because safety ranks high in our survival needs. According to modern science fear is hardwired in our biology because we live in a dangerous universe which requires ample warning before disaster befalls on us. Daoism ranks fear as three of the three root emotions from which all other emotions are created, including love and happiness. We usually feel unsafe when something happens to us that we have not experienced before. We can feel anxiety about things or even fear. In Chinese and western medicine alike anxiety and fright are seen as harmful to the heart and certainly not as a helpful factor to our decision making process. Fear and even shock are seen in Chinese medicine as destructive for concentration and thus causes the qi of our internal tissues to shoot in all directions so that we lose coherence in our behavior, or in some cases even our consciousness. In that sense modern times offer us the greatest of challenges. We have to learn to deal with modern risks and difficulties and also with how we can reinterpret the wisdom of our forefathers. Stress, burn-out syndrome and many other problems are anxiety and fear related diseases.

Our relative wellbeing gives us time to ponder over our options in life. Modern commerce uses advertisement and other form of seductive reasoning to help us spend as much of our wellbeing on buying things. People often like to not spend things on unnecessary things, but if you look in their homes, you often see many things they do not need to survive. To have these things is sign of their celebration of safety.

When we grow older we more often than not hear people complain about the missed changes in life. They often wished they knew more, were more skilled, paid more attention, were more healthy and so on. Well, that is what we learned from the past. We all know we could do so much more than average if we would put more effort in things.

In Chinese and other East Asian societies there often is a moral obligation to succeed in life. In western culture that is not seen so much as important anymore. It is seen as pleasant to succeed, but being happy and healthy often weights more than reputation. As a result relative laxness is often tolerated as a lifestyle. This laxness can lead to premature aging because of the relative inactivity of body and mind. Daoist Yangsheng follows Laozi in suggesting that we should not live a hurried lifestyle, but it also suggests that nothing should be left undone. Laozi himself suggested to live a playful lifestyle and to follow age-old experiential wisdom at the same time. What we can take from that is that thinking forward and knowing what is our plan in life can help us achieve a lot without having to be in a hurry. To do so we need to understand the natural order in our life, our aging process and the natural seasons time goes through. Our personality changes when we age, our needs change. These things do not need to be a weakness, but can be a strength when we understand them. Daoist Yangsheng suggests that our greatest strengths can be found in soft power, in our weaknesses and our errors.

In observation health we see that averageness in our health easily leads to a diffuse management of our lives. Since nothing spectacular happens to us our consciousness is oftentimes half asleep as a result of our sense of safety.

When people suffer from what Chinese medicine calls a 'xu' condition their health as a force has become partly or completely 'impoverished'. The downpart of that condition is that we feel we are plagues by all kinds of ailments. There seems to be something wrong too often, if not all the time. The upside of the condition is that we become very sensitive for all kinds of influences and in our reasoning we easily perceive how events weigh or not weigh in a supportive way to ourselves. Fear is one of the core feelings belonging to this condition. In xu conditions we often sense the fairness and unfairness of situations more easy. When untrained in regulating ourselves it can lead to worry in our thinking. We are also more quickly aware of when something goes wrong so we are possibly more on time to respond to changes.

When people suffer of a 'shi' condition we see that their health force is overly abundant. Where in literature 'xu' is associated with poverty, 'shi' is associated with opulence of yang. Technically the Huangdineijing suggest the body cannot have too much yang. Yang is here the liveliness of out body. But it also suggests that yang should be properly regulated and distributed to avoid developing disease. The downpart of shi is that we feel so strong that we easily become insensitive to other people's needs or weaknesses. Arrogance is a feeling that belongs to a 'shi' condition. Ofcourse when in a shi condition we are feeling strong enough to keep on going, at least until we have become burned out. Our shi condition makes us more insensitive to change and danger.

We see that both cases have benefits and difficulties to deal with. In fact we can note that the middle way between them has two appearances. One is the middle way of diffuse existence that is neither sensitive nor strong. The other middle way is the middle way of conscious existence which has the benefits of both xu and shi conditions, namely being both sensitive and strong. The first middle way can happen to anyone but the second middle way is an ideal middle way although it occasionally happens to people that they find themselves on that middle way, the event itself usually is only a teaser. We call it that we are on a role, or in the flow or something. It only rarely happens to people naturally. Fortunately learning is also a natural process, so by means of education and learning this state can be achieved, maintained and fine-tuned. We can work on it and play with it every moment of the day. The sensory effect is an intensification of the experience of life: we feel motivated by the awareness that life is an urging experience. Life wants to flourish, open like a flower and be involved with every event in life at the same moment. We see in this that the effort to function better can help us experience life better and create more happiness with life. An extra is that we learn to deal with our energy more efficiently as well and as a result we tend to age less fast and tend to stay young, flexible and adaptive up to a higher age, extending the good and vital times of life till more close to our death, and thus shortens our suffering in case illness happens to us before we die.

Health study is the study of qi and dao

"Dao is birthing yuanqi
Yuanqi is birthing jingyangqi and jingyinqi
Jingyangqi and jingyinqi mingle with
each other to create zhongqi[1]

---

1 Zhongqi, 中氣 means mean qi or central qi, a base qi from which things come forth. It is also how we represent ourself to others.

Zhongqi is the state where jingyin and
jingyang qi commune without conflict
Jingyangqi and jingyinqi and zhongqi are
birthing the ten thousand things
And become contained in the ten thousand things
Therefore: all things support yin and embrace yang
Opposition and unification are on friendly terms (balanced)"

The above is a retranslation from a creation myth from China. Yuanqi 元氣 means first qi, or origin qi, or where things come from. Jingyang and jingyin are both preceded by the character jing 精, which means both perfect as well as essential and skilled. It indicates the patterning of things, how they generate their existence. The first part of the character is rice. Rice is seen as a form of perfection because rice always looks the same says Karlgren in his dictionary of etymology. In qigong we commonly translate jing as 'constructive (essencial activity), based on the meaning 'skilled' and 'perfect' because being skilled also implies proficient action that makes skilled. In Chinese and Daoist medicine texts Jing is seen as originating in our kidneys, where there is a yin and a yang component is. In popular texts the meaning of jing is given as essence, as if it is a substance. But from these texts yinjing is determined as that what precedes action, which is memory, physical memory. Yangjing is an action, often seen as the weaving of the tissues of the body. Yangjing is that what generates memory. The kidneys are responsible for maintenance of body memory in Chinese medicine. Currently it is popular to see Jing as the fascia of the body, which to a degree is certainly relevant. Fascia is used in the process, but the muscles or muscle channels too. Most important is that Chinese and Daoist medicine texts make clear that jing is where the generation of health takes place. Jinmg is exercized. In food that means that what we eat primarily what makes the food itself, and that is the jing. The jing gives the animal or plant its form (xing).

it is clear that Zhongqi, 中氣 means mean qi or central qi, a base qi from which things come forth. This creation myth originates from a modern Chinese interpretation by an anonymous Chinese author. In his introduction he explains the alchemical foundation of Laozi's Daodejing use. In doing so he uses so called 'dictionary terminology'. By retranslating to original terminology to pinyin more of the original flavour of his intent is recognizable.

What is elemental in this text is the different kinds of qi being discussed, all being sub-defined by additional terminology, betraying a highly technical use of language. The concept of qi is in the story connected with two factors, namely Dao and perfection. The technical use of language also seems to contain a classification system: perfect and non-perfect implied, but also yin and yang. Both also mean Dao and not Dao. Showing us a division of four:

Jingyang	*Jingyin*
Yang	*Yin*

What we see here is a theory of 'perfection in levels' and an 'either this or that division of things'. The either this or that division of things as yin and yang seems to be continuous and have a foundation in qi and Dao as a harmonious unity. The division in layers of perfection seems to be a subdivision within each category of things. So again we might analyse the text as such:

1st layer	*Qi*
2nd layer	*Yinyang*
3rd layer	*Level of Perfection*

The combination of these layers are the foundation of what we will from here forward call the 'yin yang theory'. The Yin Yang Theory is a central concept that helped create Daoland healthsports and care programs. The Yijing counsellor course, a 2 year learning program is used to finetune that knowledge for professional use as well as indepth understanding of the root theories of Chinese and Daoist Medicine as an independent science.

In the case of our search to health, long and happy lives we may say that Dao, qi, perfection and optimal health come together. We can understand from this that health is an ongoing process that never really stops requiring activity and learning. So something like health is something we do, not something we have. In western language health is often described as a possession (have health) or identification (be healthy). In Chinese language Jiankang (health) is related to the establishment of oneself as a person. In the west the concept of health remains more ambivalent.

In most of our lives our health is something that comes and goes and hardly tried to give direction or being controlled. But when we are successful in doing things we often feel happier and also healthier. On the other hand we also see that when our health is good we feel happier to do things and that increases our chances of being successful. In this case we seem to radiate vitality, our qi is effective and thus we have Dao or we Dao (verb), which some translators translate as 'way-making' and others as 'the way'.

In Daoism Great Dao is seen as an organizing principle preceding the world we live in. although we might be insufficient in describing Dao itself, we are able to describe its effect. Its effect is the natural order of things, events and relations between things/events. When the natural order is disturbed then qi diminishes or becomes over abundant and damages the system more. If our lives are not all that natural

We seem to feel out of place with things, events and relations. It also explains why for some people disease seems to be exactly the right thing to increase their happiness and bonding with life. Health in the Daoland concept is therefore not only the absence of disease or the presence of vitality. It is mainly the establishment of a person that can maintain and develop his or her independent self in life and society without having to develop a parasitic relationship with fellow beings. Parasitic in that sense means that life is directed by a dependency. The dependency is the parasite, not the person. The dependency causes some kind of panic when the source of dependency is witheld. The panic is an emotion, and an emotion is a composit of intention driven behavior. All emotions are according to chinese medicine theory based on aversions. The three root avarsions are desire, andger and fear. All the other emotions are composits of these. So an emotional dependency automatically reveals an avarsion. The aversion usually is that what would make you in dependent, autonomous of the cause. Some people emotionally depend on medicines, others on drugs, money, power, love, sex, sports, prestige, feeling weak, feeling strong etc. The fulfillment of that dependency creates a sensation of happiness, exitement, love, etc. The dependency also creates a partial artificial lifestyle that gradually undermines our health. Art often expresses aspects of that dependency. The irony is that only we ourselves can determine if we are dependent or not, although in many cases there are also outward signs though which others can guess we have one or more dependencies. In my classes I call these dependencies usually 'crutches', things we need to appear healthy and normal. The thought processes that come with dependencies are rationalizations that clarify why it is ok to keep having that dependencies. Often these take the form of radicalization, increased beautification of the artificiality, mystification, spiritualization, holding on to opinions over facts, falsification of meanings etc. Basically most of what got our modern life into the problems piling up, and putting us as a species, and as an individual or community at risk.

In this definition having a disease is not necessarily related to having health or not. The goal of the Daoland program therefore is to create health, not to cure disease, although that might be a side effect of Disciplining and Cultivating health.

Life's habits

Someone told me once he considered life a cruel event. The Indian Prince, Gautama de Buddha 2600 years ago spoke similarly but more elaborate in that respect about the four noble truths. Of which the first one was the fact that we all suffer one way or the other. His second truth can be summarized with a sense of displeasure about this suffering. The third truth is that we can/want devise means to diminish our suffering. His fourth truth states we actually practice something to diminish suffering. The reality of both this person and the Buddha is that life is something that becomes better and more pleasurable over time if we work on it, but at times if feels like swimming against the current. The art of life is to never let go of our confidence and sense of well- being in all of the hardship. Health practice therefore also contains an element of finding pleasure in the challenges hardship offers

We can state that our lives are complex sets of truths, half-truths and false truths. Moreover, many truths we live by are only partly understood. It is arrogance from our side to consider ourselves smart or wise. For most of us our minds and feelings are a patchwork of momentary decisions, true and false memories, fantasies and unspecified moods anc feelings. The comfort of our body also is often a random events. We often induce comfort through escapist moments where we stimulate our senses in often aggressive ways to numb the feelings of dissatisfaction lingering from other activities within us. This behavior enhances our aversion of what makes us feeling bad, even if we feel bad about them for the wrong reasons. It also doesn't give us the space to understand why it makes us feel bad or prevent it from happening or using the moment better a next time. The collection of these behaviors we call 'bad habits'. An example what more and more people consider a bad habit is 'smoking'. The bad habit is not the smoking, but the smoking against better judgment. Knowing something is a bad habit but allowing this bad habit to persist undermines our vitality because we have already judged ourselves as lazy, doing something wrong, addicted or anything else we intuitively know of is not helping us. It also undermines our trust in ourselves to make the right choices in moments when it really matters. Persisting in bad habits of minor nuisance that can be easily changed and do not require excuses to stop changing them undermine our moral strength. It makes us develop vagueness/fuzziness in what we consider good or bad.

Likewise, developing a good habit and exercising the good habit to help it become second nature it thus helps us develop our vitality. Similarly it helps us define clear moral boundaries and trust in ourselves doing the right thing at the opportune moment. People become often moral relativist or rigid in their morality because they have bad habits. It takes time an effort to recognize what are good moral habits.

Laozi's advice on these things was to build a more simple lifestyle, reduce the anxieties and sense of guilt caused by doing things against better judgment. In Chinese Yangsheng the advice is similar:

- *Develop a relaxed lifestyle, but do not be passive*
- *Don't worry too much about fortune and misfortune. These things come and go. They belong to the weather of life*
- *Be patient with events and people and wait with judging them until you recognize how they support you. Prevent judging them on the basis of how you feel injured by them. Injury is often a perception, not a reality.*
- *You don't have to stop bad behaviors, but do them conscious but on the level where they do not harm you. This way you also radicalize them to the point where they become ridiculous and lose their power over you.*

These activities are called developing good habits. Make sure you are fit in multiple levels of your being, which means spend everyday time to exercise your abilities and fine-tune your skills. This is called developing good habits.

Good habits

In the following we will discuss some more good habits in which the Daoland offers tools for experience and learning:

1) Methods of nobility

One of the main contributions to worry and fear in the world is our fear for the competitive fellow beings whom might have or might not have the best intentions with our personal prospects. We have a natural trust in the goodness of people, and that is why in general we are nice people. But that trust can be shaken by many different factors. As a result it is easy to seek blame for the misfortunes of our life by others or in some cases by ourselves. Blaming others or ourselves is not helpful although it sometimes is a relieving factor to discuss the mechanisms of how things got all wrong. We all know that criticizing others and gloating about our goodness does not really contribute. Following Laozi we suggest that it is better to work on being a good example for how things can also be done. Doing the things to the best of your abilities and making sure you get better at it is enough of a comment.

2) Exercising one's self

People usually do not understand the concept of exercise. What eve r we exercise is always our self or an aspect of our self. Even if we practice only our backhand routine in tennis we exercise an aspect of our self because playing tennis is an aspect of our identity. And our identity and our self is the same. Our pains, hour hopes, desires and behaviors are all expressions of our thinking or signs of the fact that we think. In fact thinking and behavior are identical to each other. Thinking without integration in behavior is not thinking, it is losing oneself in speculation and detail. What people usually sideline as pure thought in fact is a form of self-inflation and no more than mere entertainment. It becomes only valuable if it contributes to society and nature at large. Science as such is valuable, research is valuable, philosophizing about things is valuable, but all these valuables have to fit in a greater plan. Nobody but you can see where your thoughts have to go to. Your thoughts are part of your behavior and therefore can be exercised just as the rest of your self. In the case of Daoland we talk basically about physical exercise combined with awareness and guidance training. Physical exercise is considered to be any bodily activity that enhances life's performance or maintains physical fitness and overall health and wellness. It is performed for various reasons. Some people practice for health reasons, others for a beautiful body and again others for feeling good or excelling in one's profession or love making.

But exercise does do so much more. Exercise is a compilation of trial and error, trying out abilities, mental concentration, managing emotions, developing endurance, willpower, patience, coordination, strategic insights and so on. Practice is research, not mindless repetition of a dance. Every move is every time a unique event. Every solution to an occurring problem is a unique solution only relevant at that time. Next time another pathway might have to be followed. Dao is not linear but organic. This is why eastern philosophy is not about numbers and rhythm like in the west, but about feeling the appropriateness of something to make things and relations do good work. It is also why Wudang Daoists and Shaolin Buddhists made martial arts an essential part of their spiritual training. It helps stabilizing the mind, opening oneself up to possibilities and never get tired when facing disappointment.

Well exercised people are also well balanced people. Being strong generally does that to you. But unaware strength can make your heart rigid and prevent you from adapting to the circumstances when so required. Well exercised people feel more confident making decisions and are less quick to feel regrets about lost changes and things out of control. In general we see that well exercised people have become prepared to deal with things before they actually happen or without beforehand wondering too much about what the problems might be that they come to face. When talking about problems it is time we discuss the concepts of shi-over abundance and xu- impoverished. Commonly they are translated as excess and deficient. Although these words are wrong to use in English, they are insufficient in the width of their meaning. The reason for this we find in shi and xu being concepts dealing with frequent maintenance in cultivation. They are not mechanical terms but farmer concepts and civilizational understandings, in the way we can see a building being worn out. Adding poles to support it doesn't make it better, and adding makeup or richer decorated clothes doesn't make anyone more healthy.

We could say that well exercised people automatically take a more proactive stance in life because they can afford to do so. When suffering a shi condition we easily become too rigid and cannot respond fast enough, we are overburdened by our success. When in a xu condition it is more easy to understand the problem, but maybe not have the ability to enforce decisions because we are in a too decrepit state to do reliable action.

Likewise when we are taken care of, such as in acupuncture treatment, massage or even herbal therapy we can learn methods to help the methods work better for us. We are full of natural anjd unnatural defense mechanisms which require therapists to use more forceful methods to break thought them, but which also cause much harm to our wellbeing. When we are a proactive element of any form of care service we can do with lower impact therapies, less medication and become more proud on ourselves in dealing with our problems.

So, what is an exercise? Exercise always has two parts: the exercise of a body or body part and the experience of the exercise. A well performed exercise is fully experienced, not only in its peak experience, but in the fullness of all its implications and complications. You see every event is quite an entertaining rollercoaster event, developing out of every event that preceded it. Everything we do is a stepping stone for the next thing we do and determines the quality of what we do and achieve. If you do not believe that, wake up with a hangover in the morning and you know what I say is true in everything. Likewise much of what we are is the result of the interaction between nature, society and our parents which provide a basis for what we might achieve or how we might transcend our weaknesses. You cannot blame your parents for it, but you can learn to handle yourself and your uniqueness as a gift and chance to enjoy life to the fullest. An exercise then is to show us how to get more effect out of life and have it more enjoyable too.

Because our bodies are very complex feedback and feed forward constructions we can come to learn how processes within ourselves take place, how gentle the forces of these processes often are, and how easy it is to guide these process by means of simple practices into most beneficial directions. The practice of this is neigong, internalized practice. Sometimes it is called neidan, internalized self-medication. Neigong is the art of reception and guidance. As far as Daoland is concerned neidan and neigong are an elemental part of both Chinese medicine study as well as of yangsheng practice. In fact, the whole of Chinese medicine clinical practice is based on people's self-experience. In defiance of western scientific opinions the ideology of Chinese medicine is based on superior knowledge through success in solving issues in oneself. It is said that without the skill to guide experiences and effect, no medication can have the effect it is supposed to have. Side effects from medication are the result of lack of self-knowledge and ability to self-manage of the physician and the client together. One part of the success of medicine ingestion is then how you comport yourself. How you comport yourself is the result of exercise, not of faith, divine intervention or of luck or bad luck, or at least, it shouldn't be. The same counts for food. You can eat and stuff yourself, or you can eat and absorb the food essences. The food essence is what makes the food good at being a living being, not your salad. From the moment something dies its essence withers and thus it becomes powerless. With herbs by making dry like stone a new essence is generated, that was supposed to purify and freeze some of its natural essence. Dried fruits and fresh fruits do not have the same effects on the body. But how can you validate that without proper experience?

Neigong is not easy to learn, because it takes time to do it right, not because it is very difficult. In fact in neidan practice there are several different levels of practice possible. For common health purpose just being aware of your physical and emotional/ mental processes and how common actions influence them is enough. The experience when properly guided with ideology will help you develop tools of support. It is a natural feedback and feedforward system that we are borrn with. It is our ability to be analytical and make associations between seemingly non-related events. Taking care of your food then, or talking care of your body is therefore also a learning school for how to analyze socio-political events in life and society.

Most popular nowadays are Ming dynasty based Neidan practices which mix Daoist and Buddhist ideas. These are described as strict techniques. But several people, including my shifu You Xuande have pointed out that neidan practice is a personal practice, and therefore the solutions to make it work are personal, not mechanically fixed. This does not mean that methods should become unique. The basic anatomy of experience to reach a particular goal is for every individual more or less the same. Existing Routines have proven themselves to be valid solutions within a particular ideological system. Outside that system you have no clue to what solution or problem might evolve. The way we practice routines can be very personal or maybe should be very personal as an experience, not as a form.

All people share similar forms, so practice to reach a particular goal also should be similar, not uniform. Two exact the same medical pills cannot have the same effect. It is illogical to be like that. People change throughout the day, renew body cells, shed old ones, eat different things, we are in continuous change, we are not continuous.

The actual form of practice serves as an anchor of continuity, to make sure we do not get lost in our own imaginations due to the natural process of change. Although we can all function according to the same ideal principles, we all have different origins, disfiguring our metabolism and body tensions in different ways. A therapist or teacher can therefore only understand our problems to a limited degree. It is also the reason why practice is never a mindless repeating of routines, but that every movement requires an inquisitive attention. An exercise is played and investigated while performing the exercise. The same goes for undergoing bodily service in the form of acupuncture or massage: it is experienced, played and investigated. That is the way to get the best results out of everything and to also enhance the pleasure level of what you are doing. It is also the way how children learn, and children learn the fastest. The exercises given in this book are therefore general frameworks for conveying principles which can be adapted to any form of exercise but especially to the whole set of Daoland practices and experiences. In Wudang culture of yangsheng it is summarized as: 'we all have different yuanfen, so we all have a different qi', loosely translated this means that our futures are all different so our purposes are different too. That is exactly why healthcare is your personal business: only you can master yourself.

3) To never give up on yourself

One of the most different things to deal with in life is the anger about aging and disease. Almost everyone gets annoyed at first but after some time of observing themselves age or gradually getting more sick and struggling blindly to find a way out of it gets irritated. Many get gradually more disappointed due to growing dependency on (often expensive) help. The result is that many people gradually sit life out and wait until they die. It is why life to many seems meaningless. They look for hope and strength in drugs, religion, drinking, violence, gambling, and so on.

That is a pity, because they waste a lot of time not enjoying the pleasure of doing useful things. Psychological research has shown that people when they age because of their problems keep living in their past and therefore miss opportunities to be part of the present or even the future. As a result their life gradually becomes less eventful, confirming the truth of how they have convicted themselves. Drugs, religion, drinking, violence, gambling, and so on in themselves are meaningless. If we use them as medicines we harm ourselves. If we use them as tools in the process of being good people that build the strength to support their fellow beings, then that makes them good. It is what is called doing good by means of what in itself is evil in Chinese Daoist, Buddhist and Confucian cultures.

We see that other people stay engaged with life, they exercise, travel, play games, develop their creativity, investigate art, study, maybe even take drugs, or being involved in religious practice or gongfu classes and so on up to a high age. Their mobility keeps their minds fresh and their body strong and agile. The period of suffering at the end of life seems more bearable, shorter on dependency and bigger on pleasure.

What the Daoland program takes from this is that it is never too late to restore one's vitality and exercise one's ability to enjoy life. Our tools, from the facial massage and acupuncture renovation and vitalization treatments to the healthsports classes: they all aim to serve as a stepping stone to excellence from whatever level you start. When starting older people often object to the Wudang fitness classes. But after some period of regaining vitality entering wudang fitness classes is a natural step, and also a personal victory marker over the aging process and one's earlier passive violation of one's self.

It is never a good time to give up on yourself. Your body, mind, life can always be rebooted and upgraded, if not to perfection, then at least to a gradual improvement that brings joy and hope in life. Your skin can look vibrant to high age, your joints can be well lubricated and your muscles can remain elastic and with firm grip to a high age.

The secret of being able to keep becoming younger over time or to stay young when you start early with a program like this is to not force your progress. Let a program naturally evolve, build in variation and study moments. Don't hesitate to ask a Daoland master for advice, even if it is only through email. Never hesitate to compare your result with fellow Daoland citizens. Share your reports on the net or in the healthclub for staffers ton process it and read the reports that others share with you. Comment on each other and be truthful and considerate.

Exercise is much about developing consciousness. Everyone who does sports has to take care of several aspects: making the most out of your movement is one, but also preventing damage, maintaining balance and planning ahead. Most modern sports do not support sportspeople enough to avoid damage completely. People who professionally sport often pay for their profession long after their body is incapable of doing more sports. The cause of this is that modern sports tries to emulate events on the battle field and on a battle field you either survive or you die. How you survive is not that important.

In Daoaland sports and care programs likewise we as users are trained to become conscious of what is happening during practice and being massaged or receiving acupuncture. But where in regular sports parts of the body are over emphasized to be able to perform, in Daoland Healthsports and care programs every time the whole body is taken in consideration, and thus in every practice consciousness is spread out over the whole body. The end result is not a preparation for struggle, but the struggle was to prepare you for better performance in life. So, the whole body is practiced as part of behavioral needs. This skill is taken from Wudang Taijiquan, where force is guided through the whole body and taken from the relation of our weight with the ground.

Fighting is nothing but a metaphor of how we behave in our actions. If we stop struggling we can start performing and improving. Within the Taiji movements all the body parts are grinded into rotation to work independently and jointly in creating strength. At the same time we minimize muscle effort by paying attention to maximize the relaxation of our muscles as a means to make the use of our muscles more efficient. We also develop continuous stretch in our movements to make sure the blood flow and channelqi flow remains alert and regular. This helps keeping our body clean of waste products, our breath even and our mind calm. Even in fast moving exercise, such as in our Wudang Fitness program.

In animals we often see that their strength seems to supersede their relative insignificant body content or shape, such as ants. But an ant can carry 6x his body weight. In retarded people we also often see a larger strength then to be expected from lack of exercise but which is due to less consciousness controlled body movements. It shows that the mind can help us as much that it acts as a break on our performance. It also shows that much of what we can and cannot do is due to inhibitions. Our fears, anger, desire and other feelings control us and limit us, but so do the things we believe about ourselves. So for healthsake self help in healthcare means braking down much of our ideas about ourselves. And that is why cultural ideologies are so important. They can show us our possible abilities. Modern culture suggest that what we see is the ideal by means of statistics, so from what we need for health we understand that can only be a misguided form of thinking.

Science itself does not believe in that idea. Science itself acknowledges the ideal situation of things as a possibility. It is our own human laziness that has made the system into this passive form of self-mutilation through permitted dependency and decay. For us in Daoland health care we wish to learn to guide our strength and relaxation to allow our body to develop its natural possible power without being too much limited by the mental effort to control the details of our abilities by our belief system that is based on what we have seen from others. Our belief system is what tells us what we can and what we cannot do. The purpose of our training program is also to help you investigate the borders of your belief system, to learn where we limit ourselves and to learn where we can develop and grow.

When we exercise we can achieve results in two ways:

1. *The pathway of Excessive Force. You can go to the limits of your achievements and cross these limits. This is called the pathway of haste. It damages your muscles and causes acidification due to increased muscle waste levels, stress responses and production of endorphins in your blood that do not only have an addictive effect, they cause what is called a Pavloff Cascade that requires you to be in panic frequently to get your shot of happy*

chemistry. In some books this is called the 'Fire method' or 'Military method'. It is the application of agression and violence to the body. It sees the body that needs to be subdued. It divides you in two classes of being: the 'I' and the 'Body/Slave/Object'. The I only sees of the body what it wants to see: its successes and failures.

2. *The pathway of patience is the method where you go to your limits and remain in a residential consciousness close to your limits. You make the presence in this area of your capacity limits into comfort zone by habitually returning there. Because of that your capacity limits gradually shift away further so that your achievements increase. It is where the 'I' and 'Body' work together and integrate. Your muscle become more moist and the metabolic rate of your tissues remains organized, which means that waste products are safely transported away, you stay relaxed and do not produce muscle rigidity as a result of acidification. You will still create a pleasant feeling, but it is much more clearheaded then the one caused by endorphins. In some books this is called the . Water method' or 'Civil method'. It dissolves the boundaries between 'that what wants' and 'that that acts'. This union is negotiating its future between the needed and the timline to reach the set goals.*

The truth is ofcourse that sometimes fire is good, but only to enhance the power of water. Many engines use the principle of combining fire under water. In Chinese medicine this is seen as the interaction between the warm heart and the wet kidneys. Together they casue teh water of the body to get heated and like central heating warm the body and allow it to live. It is in Chinese and Daoist medicine te core quality of yin and yang that motivates our youthfulness, or when it fails our aging and formation of disease.

The pathway of patience is not difficult to follow, but it is important to not slip away from the area of your limits. If you slack a bit too much you drive your limits down. You cool down in an effort to maintain your warmth. But you aklso decrease your ability to circulate the warmth and nourish your body parts, resulting in slowing down and wrinkling. Like when you have a stiff neck and you prevent it from moving. As a result your muscles have the risk to remember the pain or tension as a good thing with as a result that you in fact limit your movement capacity. As all practice it requires self-discipline to not forget your goals. If you do, you set the clock on aging. Living therefore makes you the janitor of your life and your body. Self cultivation in DIY Healthcare, and thus autonomy, means you un derstand what you need to do, and you actually do it.

One goal of the Daoland program is to avoid what most sports and care programs do wrong, namely to let you specialize in your achievements:

- *Sport often lets you force shortterm gains for long term trauma/damage*
- *Care programs often focus on the ability of certain muscles, and not on the systemic cultivation of full ability.*

This program advocates a more generalized process. It was first mentioned in the Daodejing, by Laozi. It said that specialization is causing problems, and that general living helps to live longer and happyer. It doesn't mean that lack of development is healthyer, it means that developing onzelf more boradly is better than emphasis on specifics. How e realize this? First of all by actively participating in the Research and/or the Daoland program as a person and not as a body or mind; Secondly by allowing natural progression through the achievements of your body. Although it is suitable to be alert and investigative during practice, it is also good not to get stuck in one type of sports for too long a time. Usually to improve on a particular sport for 2 to 6 months is advisable, then switch to another practice in the program and repeat participation every-now-and-then the earlier sports so that skill keep on developing and your stamina in that particular fitness remains on track. How much repeat can differ from person to person. Eventually you find yourself rotate through different sports. In our research we investigate the truth of this by setting people up in different combinations of learning the three core programs of food medicine, meditative awareness and gongfu fitness. I selected these three for the program because as a combination they cover many fields of activities that you need to generate 'foundational health'.

As I clarified this program as a DIY Healthcare coincides with Laozi's advise not to specialize oneself as part of the Dao to live longer and more healthy. The application of Laozi's thoughts in sports and medicine focuses on working with the capacity to be healthy, and not necessarily with the details of disease causing factors. The wisdom of this is that in managing the whole of our body we put our discomfort causing factors back to the relative position within the body to help ourself reintegrate these factors in the natural order of our body. As Laozi says: Dao is never far away. The Dao of health is just as near. It is also from this that we can draw the meaning of being natural, not as being just as one is at the moment, but being what is one's capacity.

PART 6

Daolands manual for the human geometry of life

This chapter wants to be a succinct as possible. In fact it gives away the secrets of health and how it is applied in Daoland programming. These are details derived from Chinese Taiji Gongfu and Qigong practice, but after comparison with ideas from other cultures on principles of health, if they had such an idea on the physical level. The origin of many peoples in the world originates health in behavior. Very few original ways of thinking link health to the body alone. Even modern medical science relates belief-system to health. All trust in a belief-system is gnostic in nature, which means you cannot know the truth of something before you have tried it and given yourself time enough to see results. The below items will help you to improve your general health. You will still need healthy exercises, and ofcourse I advice to involve yourself one way or another with Daoland programs.

- *Size matters: maximize your form*
- *The Dao of straightness*
- *The Dao of roundness*
- *Daoland principles of joint position*
- *The root of breath*
- *Apply in daily life and sports*

1 Size matters: maximize your form

Many people tend to slope their back and shoulders or be tight and rigid. These minimize the size of your body form. Pay attention especially when you are tired

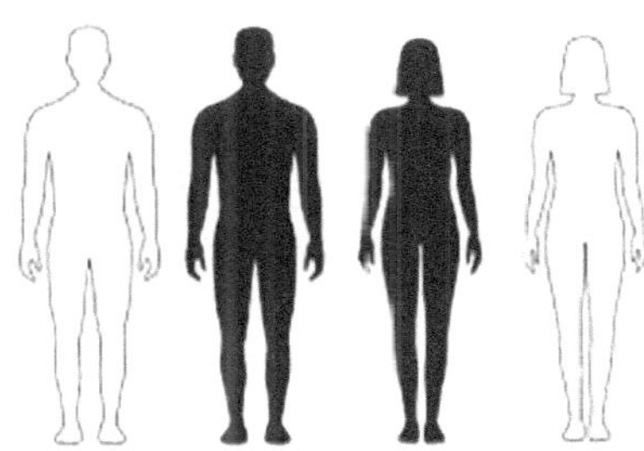

to maximize your body form. This means you try to take up as much space as you can so that the content volume of your body is maximized. The maximum volume allows your inner factory to do its job better and produce better quality nourishment out of the things you eat, drink and breathe or talk about.

The foundation of this process is found in the activity of the 养精-Yangjing we talked about before. Yang means life, or development. Yang is from 养生-yangsheng, the cultivation or development of growth. The yangjing generates yang. Yang is the warmth and activity of the body. Yang is the process of generating Jing. It also requires attentive awareness, for which the Chinese name is 神 shen. Your awareness is required to finetune. Growth without guidance is like a tumor. It doesn't go anywhere useful.

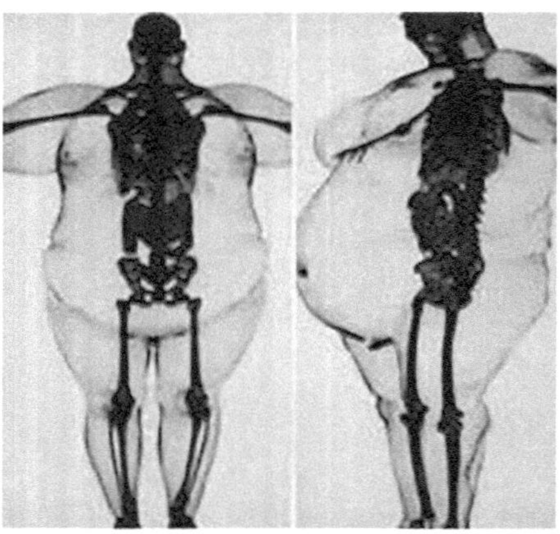

Of course, maximizing your inner volume excludes growing white fat and thus enlarging the hulk of your body. When you grow white fat in fact you shrink in functional space. Fat clots the interstices between cells and thickens cell walls (which are made of fatty tissue too) and reduce the capacity of your body to nourish itself. Fat also slows down your awareness and puts a serious resistance in your movement.

White fat is caused by cooling down of yang before it reached its goal, and from overconsumption of foods and drinks the body has no time to digest, or that are things it puts on a long line for digestion, such as soda's, meat, transfats etc. Accumulation of white fat causes systemic overweight. I like to make clear that overemphasized bulging muscles also contain more water than useful (fat is condensed yang-water), therefore i also like to put them in the category of excessive weighjt or overweight. Overweight people suffer continuous friction in their body, like as if you are in doubt of acting. BMI standards are based on acceptable overweight. True health and natural fitness takes place slightly below these standards of weight. Overweight, -however practical for cold cold winters when moderate fat- is a nuisance for your health.

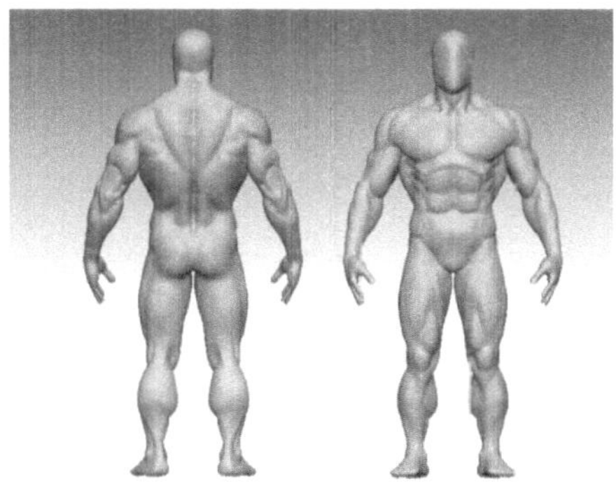

Do not forget: feeling/ being tired or stressed is not a reason to slack in controlling yourself, they are the reason why you ought to increase control of yourself. Real exercise only takes place when you are tired or stressed, and not when you are rested, feel comfortable and happy. Being tired or stressed are the limits of your fitness. This is where you need to stretch your boundaries by developing gradual improvements through discipline, but without stepping over your boundaries.

This is why the time-limits on Daoland practices are set as they are. The body has natural cycles of fitness and tiring. They naturally alternate during the day and practice in sets of about 25 minutes. This coincides with about 4 rotations of blood in your body and thus one set of commands for correction or decay. When you alternate Daoland activities every hour you never grow tired because your body is for every class performing other routines, allowing for development of a wider scope of general fitness. You can even allow for more change from day to day, because the body learns to increase maintenance efficiency, improves nourishment and waste cleaning due to the increased inner space on every level. In Daoland classes you will hear remarks on maximizing your inner space very frequently to remind you of maintaining maximum body form and coherence.

2 The Dao of straightness

Our body is a double bill of sensory equipment and chemical processing power. Our most important thoughts are about not immediately dying, so our alertness is a very important part of our health. Being drowsy, moody or obsessive are states that limit our consciousness and therefore help us getting more sick, weak or stressed. Because of maintaining straightness in what we do we help maximizing our awareness. By not using cushions when we sleep and sleeping on our back we also extend our consciousness into our sleep. Dreaming is healthy, but actively guiding your dreams through half sleep is better. Your life is a meditation on maintaining life. Straightness here refers to the outer general appearance of the body due to the fact that the natural curvature of the spinal column and neck

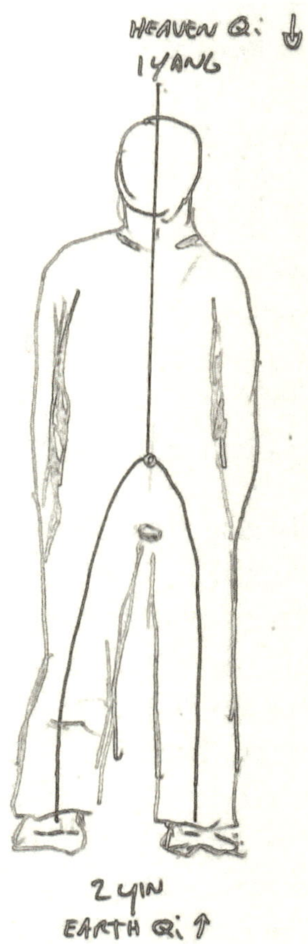

are such set that from tailbone to crown is one set straight line, allowing the maximums stretch on the spinal cord, causing it to warm the outer nerves along the spinal collum, increase regrowth of bone set capillaries, and what in Chinese medicine is called the flow of yang-steam along the dumai channel, which is in fact the ridge of dinosaur like protrusions we so often see in people with distorted back shapes. The practice is the foundation for what in Chinese alchemy is called 'successful circulation of the small cycle of heaven', referring to the dream of everlasting life, just like heaven is everlasting, straight, double and square, as the classic oracle Yijing puts it.

The straightness of the body is caught by the feeling of reaching up with the crown to heaven and sinking down with your weight in yout heals. Another aspect of that is that Chinese medicine biology from the past used to see the bones as hanging in the muscle channels, and not as in the western biological sciences as the muscles mechanically hanging on the bones. This difference in principles has consequences. One of them is the principle of Jing, the active shaping of the body. A third method is called the 'opening of the three gates'. The three gates are called the windgate at the bottom of the skull, the stone gate under the fifth throratical vertebrea, and the water gate or life gate between the kidneys and behind the umbillicus. These points can be lifted with your attention and intention, allowing the other vertrebrae to hang on them and thus relaxing the muscles and making space to free up pressure from the nerves.

Lifting the windgate relaxes neck and sholders and closes the 7th vertebra, through which the yang can be properly dispersed in the yang channels at the coloured side of the arms and along the body to the feet. It also allows for the baihui, hundred meeting point on the crown of the head to come to the top of the head. Normally it is behind the top and a bit lower. At the same time the lifting of the skull tuck in the chin in a natural way, in stead of tucking in the chin as people often are learning from amateur meditators, which in fact locks the neck. Another aspect is that the lifting of the skull allows the opening of the throatpoint at the top of the chestbone, where the condens of the body ought to be collected to go back to the kidneys along the main yin channel. Regulating the yin ua the most important function of posture.

The stone gate behind the heart and between the shoulder blades are what we can call the blocking of perception in the heart, or the blocking of the free flow of our feelings. The shoulder blades are what in Chinese medicine is called the Stone Gate, and the pericardum in modern TCM. In modern Chinese medicine it is identified with the Pericardium fleese around the heart because they couldnt make sense out of the percardium as an organ due to the superficiality of their knowledge. You have tro understand that just a fraction of original works of Chinese medicine and cultivation have been translated in western languages. That is like describing a building by means of a door, or a blind person describing an elephant by knowing one of its legs.

Another aspect of the lifting of the stone gate is the relaxation of the liver and the diaphragm, whcih for chinese medicine originally are the same. In daoism it is described as the luch meadows where children play, but it is also called the area where the army camps. The army is the blood of the body. In the Yijing (weft of exchanges, also known as I Ching), there is mention of the army camping on the left or camping on the right. It means that left or right parts of the body is troubled. Armies are sometimes at war with themselves, and thus tightening the diaphragmatic area, heating up and bothering lungs, heart, stomack or spleen/ pancreas. Soldiers are not reliable friends. They need to be pampered and kept innocent. Many revolutions in countries happen due to upset armies. So by lifting the stone gate the diaphragm is relaxed, releasing tension on the breath and agitation from the mind. It also improves anxiousness by relaxing the stomach.

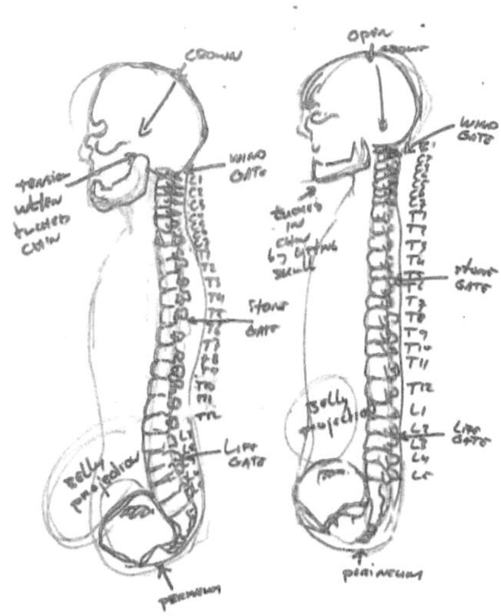

The water gate or life gate is the point where in daoist alchemy the heart fire heats up the kidney water. That water circulates through the Du and Ren vats as steam and condense. The Du and Ren are not channels, they are like lakes or vats/containers for storage. The Du runs through the spikes of your spinal collumn. The Ren over the front midline of your body. The Du and ren connect below through the perineum. The level of presumed water in the ren presses water in the dumai, and when the water meets the mingmen or life gate, it ought to be steamed up apropriately to make the body yang through its warmth. The dumai above meet through the stomach channel bridging the distance from the du to the ren through the water in the eyes. The eyes collect the condense from the crown and drips it in the ren/stomach connection. What stays in the stomach channel calms your stomach fluids, and what goes into the renmai accumulates to put pressure on mingmen. This is the mechanism of life. A bit complicated it is. Moreover, if the mingmen point is closing we become less mobile. If it is closed we basically are death. So you see that mobility is the secret to living and health.

3 The Dao of roundness

Nature works through indirect action. Heaven, God or Spirits never talk to people for the simple reason that nature doesn't understand straightness. Heaven is the only force working using straightness. That means that heaven comes down in a straght line. If it gets disrupted due to a hindering factor, it splinters and dissolves. People are able to cause that disruption in meditation. The idea that we can directly handel heaven qi is what in daoism is considered historically a herisy. In the Yijing heaven is represented by 6 dragons flying in one direction only. There is always only one point of heaven above you. Like a shower you can have it enter you, but if you are not straight and punctual you will splinter it and it is no use to you. You will not be a proper recepticle. Confucians saw themselves as representing the 'Will of Heaven', so for appropriate status they forced themselves to move in straight lines and angles. The rest of nature is different. Animals and plants eat with caution (except when extraordinary hungry) because they have to remain vigilant. They move in curls, spirals and circles to avoid detection. Even hunters do that. Daoists see straightness as for the naïve people who think being forceful and being in a hurry is a natural state. So in daily life pay attention that you move along arcs and spirals and pay attention. Make sure your body shape follows its natural patterns. It is stragiht in its vertical axis, but round in everything else. What does that mean? It means that the natural curves of your body and body parts has yang sides withc or curved outward, where the inside is curved inward. Look at your foot or hand. That is the best representative of natural roundness. The chest is the hollow inside of your chest, while your back is a slightly curved outside. This does not mean you should bend-over and keep your shoulders inward. It means that your arms naturally tend to move inward and not backward. It also means that force in your arms originates between your shoulder blades and in an outward push, not in an inward pull. The same goes for your hips. Your legs spiral outward away from the sacral bone area and not form the hip joints. Our muscles are set spiralwise to the bones. In the Daoland exercises and even the massages these principles are continuously maintained. They help to generate a natural order of the body parts that feels strong and competent. As a wake up standing exercise every morring you can reset the natural forms of your body and every day reset the aging clock of your body.

4. Daoland principles of joint position

Our joints are the breaking points of our body as any martial artist knows. Zhuangzi emphasized that joints are hollow spaces when he was talking in his stories about a butcher using Dao to slaughter cows and thus never blunt his knife. Laozi said that hollow spaces are the hub that makes a wheel. Likewise in our body the joints make our body so incredibly useful.

Our joints are encapsulated by many smaller bands of muscles. All our muscles derive their flexibility by a chemical called elastine. This elastine makes it possible that if movement warms these smaller muscles these muscles can swell and push the joints open, thus enlarging the inner space of the body significantly and allowing to make movements outwardly pushed arcs of power and not inwardly pulled retractions. It also makes it possible to use muscles and contra muscles in unison instead of alternating and thus doubling our strength while making less of an effort. Two other benefits this way of holding the joints is that the rotation space for your joints becomes larger and the regrowth of cartilage and its lubrication is stimulated. It also shows why in the for instance Daoland Wudang fitness we pay so much attention to quick joint rotations, so that the mobility of the body is stimulated. In bamboo formula qigong rotation also plays a major role, and all taijiquan is based on continuous rotations of joints and muscles.

Both Chinese Buddhism and Daoism speak of Buddha's or spirits living in the joints, allowing for a level of conscious action. Al living creatures have a natural need for space. When we put them in a too narrow space they are not only unhappy, but their health also degrades. You see this with animals being kept for consumption. Their pens are usually smallish so that a relative small space can house many animals. They are being fed fastly so that they produce a max in milk, meat or eggs in the most uneconomic way. The consume huge amounts of food and water to let them suffer from overy unnatural growth, restricted mental-emotional growth, and physical mobility to staisfy the desires of people, and at the expense of the environment and large parts of the population that live in scarcity, if not outright hunger. When Your joint are placed in a natural position you will see that the body requests less food due to increased bodily happiness and efficiency. When the joints are made tight, such as in many modern sports, we create friction and request more fuel for the work we are required to do in the tasks that we have. So we like loose joints, but also not too loose. The bones have to be sringed together, like pearls on a necklace. There should be wiggling space to move the bones together without causing friction and damage of the catrilage that covers the bones.

5 The root of breath

According to Chinese medicine when we breathe we breathe the moral impetus of heaven and according to western biology we breathe gasses. What this difference means is that the experience of breath as a consciousness-event is as important as the chemical process.

In biology breathing is seen as a reflex movement, but even if that is true that does not mean we cannot control our breathing patterns. In fact modern sports follow yoga and taiji sports in organizing their breath. And breath control follows feeling patterns which shape both the resulting effect of breath as a experiential sequence as well as the efficiency of our breathing by gradually altering the neural pathways for our lungs use. But Chinese medicine extends the workings of the lungs way beyond the biological limitations we so easy accept. It says that the cause for breathing is a feeling like hunger originating in the belly. If we eat food it is harder to feel. If we eat until we are filled we cannot feel it at all. This root of breath is a fragile feeling which is easily distorted by feelings such as fear, anger and desire, but also by other feelings. As a result of these feelings we breath more than we need, because of the fear to be short, the anger that it is not good enough and the desire not to hurt/ die. By slightly holding our breath and regulating the intake and release of breath when the belly asks for it by means of slow, thin breathing, we gradually start breathing in patterns suitable to the body. A suitable breathing pattern eliminates much of our anxieties, makes us feel more easily content and also allows for better functional nourishment and empowerment of our body, without having to rely on the oxygen expenditure that people usually adhere to. Oxygen based burning processes are hot and produce many toxins. By regulating the burn we generate more durable power. Breathing then can be a control mechanism for the body, and controller is exactly what it is being called in Chinese medicine. In the Daoland course for learning meditation much emphasis is being paid to this experiential process as to help you fine- tune your energy usage, reduce food and breath intake and slimming your load of fatigue moments.

6 Apply in daily life and sports

These 5 aspects should be applied every day in as much of your daily life as possible. In fact they are exercises for inside exercises and in fact they will help you not only to have more health and exercise results, but they will also help you make much more sense out of all the health talks you find in popular books, on tv or the internet. Information is very important, but having a way to see the relevance of information is much more relevant. Daoland provides that. It provides a rationale and a handle to deal with health and information, because that is what we are: we are bags of sense organs and processing organs. Our consciousness serves us to live as long as heaven and earth. We cannot do without movement, information and food. This is why we start our life with asking questions as part of our play, and that is what we should continue all our life.

The idea is that exercise takes place on three levels:

1. The formal exercise. Formal exercise is based on the interaction between bones and muscles to move our limbs. Usually these exercises use the large muscles, and focus on hand eye and foot hand, or foot eye co-ordination in relationship to strenght, balance and agility. These muscles are good for unrefined movements, and do not have an optimal activity economy. But they are easy to make conscious. They require large amounts of blood and nourishment to function, especially for high intensity training, forcing the body to overfeed all the time on harmful food substances, containing large amounts of stress hormones (of animal sources).
2. The princial exercise. Principle exercise uses principles of movement and uses for this largely the ligaments and minor muscles. These minor muscles help keeping

the joints friction free so that cartrilage doesn't get damaged or that it can be repaired. These minor muscles easily hold tension which will limit your joint rotation, so exercising the joint rotation as we do in the Wudang gongfu fitness program is very helpful to release these tensions. This is important because this type of muscle tension easily locks in emotional states and emotional memories, more even than the fascia do, since the fascia support habitual movement and posture, which is generated by the minor muscles.

3. In common exercises movements are usually generated by contracting muscles. In the principles of Wudang Taiji gongfu movement we use both consciously extencing and contracting the bigger and smaller muscles. This creates the opportunity to produce larger strength with less effort by using less muscle fibers, or when you do exercise the opportunity to generate more full use of muscles in a more integrated and co-ordinated, economic way.

The reason why I determine certain muscles as economic and others as less economic has to do with nourishment. Chinese medicine and Biomedicine are not fully in accord with each other.

Chinese medicine as originating in Daoism is rooted in the idea of eating only what you need, which results in all practicality intyo sort of a continuous half fast. The habit of people in China is to eat a lot, untill they sweat. The idea is to eat to overflowing you can warm your body. It is the habit of the northerners and greedy hunger that hjas taken over all of Chinese culture. But the medicine idea is that eating small bits is more easy to digest and learn from the food how to maximize the effect of food. Food is medicine. What we call medicine is extra strong food, or superfood.

Medicine should only be taken in absolute emergency. The firsty solution should come from adapting your diet and exercise regimen. To be able to do this we need to develop awareness, awareness is sometimes translated as mindfulness, but in the west it is often focussed on emotions. Awareness, or 神 shen is more a general mindfulness, or being aware of everything at the same time and the tool we need to develop our body posture (性-xing) through the composing or constructing activity (精-jing) of the body itself, using our connuction with the earth by means of our body weight and the reaction force from that weight on the ground. This is a simple feat of physics. The physics formula is $F^a = F^r$, and the reactive force is sometimes called Earth qi and sometimes called yangjing. Earthqi is not dependent on what comes from the earth, but how dense or swompy the ground under our feet is. The idea of daoist science is that the bodily ability is altering when we travel from place to place, and exercising in different kinds of landscapes is therefore important for our achievement in exercises. This is one of the topics for Fengshui studies. Fengshui isn't only for finding proper places for graves, but also for proper places to practice.

Another aspect that Daoists find important, isn't only the way how we exercise and move our body, or the place where we practice, but also that every moment is the preparation for the next. This also means that the development of alertness and the application of exercise principles in our daily actions is essential. Every thing we do, like washing dishes, doing shopping, breathing, eating, having a meeting; Everything is practice on the path to health and immortality. Taking in consideration that every lifestyle except our modern convenience style is more labor intensive, there is plenty of opportunity to practice ourself in what we do by doing more walking, or by our own handywork than through a machine. In these activities we can apply the principles, thus creating more awareness of, and coherence in our body.

The principle of exercising in Chinese medical culture is called Dao Yin (导引). Over time, this type of exercise has been widely applied to medical treatment and health preservation since ancient times, and it is also acknowledged as an effective traditional orthopaedic therapy by both ancient and modern traditional Chinese medicine. "Dao" (导) means to guide qi, the internal reflection of ones organic functioning of the body, so as to create an internal balance, and "Yin" (引) means to stretch the body so as to gain strength and flexibility. This is where we find the above described principles of movement. Through physical movements, practicing Dao Yin exercise can create the harmony of qi and blood in the body, thus achieving the purpose of preventing disease, improving health and accelerating the recovery of limb function. Dao Yin is a kind of body exercise that involves breathing, massaging through stretching and twisting arms and legs, and mental focus which act together to direct the internal messaging of the body leading to local proper functioning. When doing daoyin as a seties we call it qigong. Qigong usually has a fixed order. Qigong is using symmetry to order the body. In taijiquan the exercises are asymmetric. All of them use repetition to discipline the body and generate organic pressure to incrementally alter and improve your body. We can see that Dao Yin exercise has a broad and a narrow meaning. In the naroow meaning, as the forerunner of the so-called "dynamic exercise" developed by later generations, Dao Yin centers on body exercise supplemented by breathing and mental training, which is considered as "Dao Yin exercise". In the broad sense, any active Chinese exercise theory or method that aims to achieve the "harmony between the internal direction of channel content and external stretching of the body" can be considered as a form of "Dao Yin exercise." This can be practiced through Tu Na (expiration and inspiration), body stretching, massaging, Lian Dan (inner alchemy), Zuo Chan (sitting in meditation), inward contemplation, and so on.

These methods are habitually categorized into "Dao Yin" and "Xing Qi (promoting the circulation of qi)" in line with the traditional standards in ancient times. Both "Dao Yin" and "Xing Qi" take the cultivation of Jing (the fundamental activity which maintains the functioning of the body), qi, and body spirits (as fragments of shen-awareness) as their core, but they require different proportions of these three elements. Laying a foundation for the so-called "static exercise" developed by later generations, Xing Qi is mainly based on breathing exercises aided by body and mental training to correct asymmetries caused by any kind of tensions. Besides that it also serves as a safeguard to maintain health over time. Health gradually developes, but also degrades gradually.

7 Exercise and Aging

When we observe our life, the general opinion is that when born we are helpless, when growing up we gain capacity to do things, and when aging we become more helpless again. In the historical past most people mostly exercised by doing their tasks in life. Exercise in the European and Middle eastern Middle Ages varied by social class and was often integrated into daily life, work, or military training rather than separate fitness routines. Peasants engaged in sports and games, while knights and monks performed exercises for strength and combat readiness, such as lifting heavy stones, wrestling, and javelin throwing. Common medieval exercises included running, jumping, and using heavy objects for strength training. Understanding of the body and its needs was not common. It was very purpose directed to win a prize or to survive on the battle field. Since that time knowledge about the body is ofcourse grown in many ways. In these middle ages the sport was community oriented, while nowadays it might still be a social event but primarily it is now a vanity event or and ego satisfaction program. We do not speak of sports persé anymore, but also about exercise.

Etymologically the concept of exercise is not always very well understood outside the range of linguists. Half way the fourteenth century, exercise did mean "condition of being in active operation; practice for the sake of training." The word originates from Old French "exercice"in the 13th century: "exercise, execution of power; physical or spiritual exercise," and from the Latin exercitium "training, physical exercise" (of soldiers, horsemen, etc.). In the text before we did speak of military prqactice and civil practice. Although we often hear about Martial Arts as exercise coming from East Asia, In this part of the world there is military training, and self-cultivation, where development from professional, social and spiritual growth often is emphasized. Confucians for instance were not allowed to exercise martial moves, but they did do practices to keep their health and sanity in tact. As far as Daoism is concerned exercise is to deal with the different stages in life. For instance to prepair for pregnancy, or to improve onés skill in a job, or to deal with disease. In Daoist Chinese medicine the general idea is that exercise serves to learn how we functionas a being, but also to deal with defects. In general people can have all kind of diseases. To deal with all these details is often described as inner alchemy: dealing with the different components of self to let the immortal self emerge. For this purpose exercise serves to keep one healthy, and to delay aging, stop aging, or reverse aging. Disease is possible through accident, but is more likely due to disharmony in our composite knowable self, allowing for the formation of disease (shortterm and longterm disease).

The beneficial effects of exercise are recognized for preventing physical and cognitive decline during the aging process. However, there is still a gap concerning recommended intensity, volume, frequency and mode of exercise especially for older people. When the body has been neglegted or exercised on basis of over-use or over-burden aging is casued by wrong self cultivation and that makes that we can do less and less when aging. In this book a lot of attention is given to prevention and restoration exercises.

In 'The history of "Exercise Is Medicine" in ancient civilizations', Charles M Tipton (2014) wrote that in 2007, the American College of Sports Medicine, with endorsement from the American Medical Association and the Office of the Surgeon General, did launch a global initiative to mobilize physicians, healthcare professionals and providers, and educators to promote exercise in their practice or activities to prevent, reduce, manage, or treat diseases that impact health and the quality of life in humans. Emerging from this initiative, termed "Exercise Is Medicine", has been an extensively documented position stand by the American College of Sports Medicine that recommended healthy adults perform 150 min of moderate dynamic exercise per week. We recommend daily mild practice of about 50 minutes for optimal health and health improvement and 150 minutes spread out over 5x 30minutes for maintenance. The Daoist idea is that two factors play a role in exercise: 1) time, and 2) stamina. When doing mild exercise and one can spread one's stamina or vitality out over a longer time, that will give better long term results than doing exercise for a short time more intensive. Burst of exercise are done with less attention, they generate a rush, but also inadvertedly makes one prone to accidents and damage over time.

Physiotherapists live from people who either exercise too intensive or from people who do not do enough exercise. The

Daoland Healthbuilding aim is to never need assistance from a paramedic due to the self regulation achieved by combining meditation and exercise, as well as exercise, meditation, and nourishment. The benefit of that is that you are more aware of the changes inside your composite self, but also where these happened, how these happened, and how to reverse them instead of patching them. The result therefore is less physical trauma, and thus less slowing down and therefore healthyer aging. Does this make sense to you?

This Chinese model does not stand on its own. Zhuangzi mentioned similar principles about 600 bc.

Zhuangzi relates to exercise through the concept of "acting without action" (wei wu wei), where physical activity becomes a spontaneous, natural and fritionless process rather than a struggle. Laozi emphasized something similar, saying that his method of doing things was easy to comprehend but difficult to follow. The goal was to exercise without specializing in a particular skill as to not invite trauma and aging. He called this "form being formless" (xing wu xing).

In 2007 Tipton suggested in 'Susruta of India, an unrecognized contributor to the history of exercise physiology': 'When considering the history of exercise physiology, authors begin with Hippocrates and the "Golden Age" of Greece before mentioning Galen and the contributions from Rome. However, this approach has omitted the information from the ancient civilizations of India which flourished before and during the emergence of Mycenaen cultures. Specifically ignored have been 1) the tridosa doctrine (humoral theory), which as early as 1500 B.C., emphasized that disease occurred because of a displacement of one or more of the three humors, with health being achieved when the humors were in equilibrium and 2) the perspective of Susruta (Sushruta) who was a 600 B.C. physician who included exercise in his prescriptions to prevent and treat diseases.

Susruta not only advocated exercise to maintain equilibrium among the humors, notably kapha, he promoted exercise to minimize the consequences of obesity and diabetes. To be effective, exercise had to be daily and moderate in intensity and never excessive or to exceed the half-maximum limit for exhaustion, because disease or even death could ensue'. In our program for both the research as the full Yangsheng Bachelor level program we likewise emphasize based on Daoist traditions that exercise should never be exhaustive, but should be practiced in such a way that you can stretch out the time of practice before you reache your boundaries. Thus habit formation creates awareness of one's ability, but also a gradual shift in your ability to allow you to do more. Daoists generally point to the perspiration factor. Sweating is seen as a loss of yang, vitality, and thus should be prevented. You can allow warmt as a result of exercise to build up to a degree where sweating doesn't occur. If you cool down suddenly also isnm't seen as good, becasue the yang in or under the skin can dampen out and no longer move, giving the beginning of the formation of white fat under the skin. White fat -we know- is the accumulation of sticky water inside a fatty encapsulating wall of a cell. That cell can grow endlessly as obese people proof. So it is clear that passive lifestyles and overeating are not at all the only casues of overweight. But what is c;lear is that daily mild exercise helps you to control your vitality and your weight, But you need a complete approach with meditation, proper nourishment and exercise in a way where these are tailered to each other in one verarching theory. This is where I have to refer to the research which I will later explain more about and where I hope you will come to participate in.

I want to also highlight the negatives of inactive lifestyles. My own parents are an example of that and I have always regretted I was never able to motivate them to do some exercises. Fortunately I am not alone in emphasizing exercise against inactivity. A series highlighting the physiological and pathophysiological bases and consequences of physical inactivity was originally proposed by the Journal of Applied Physiology Editor Jerome Dempsey. The plan was to present a survey of a number of the organ systems/ functions/diseases (blood vessels, central circulatory function, cognitive function, death, metabolism, nonalcoholic fatty liver disease, and skeletal muscle) that are affected by physical inactivity. Bed rest, reduced daily stepping, and a sedentary, inactive lifestyle were highlighted as experimental models. The aim was to provide insights into biological mechanisms by which physical inactivity leads to dysfunction and negative health consequences. This is abasically also the above mentioned BA level Yangsheng program.

A common assumption is, that physical inactivity merely is the reverse of exercise training. For example, in resistance vessels, physical inactivity results in upregulation of vasoconstrictor pathways, rather than affecting vasodilator function. This is the proces of tightening or widening of blood vessels. It is also found in research that compared with a physically active group, an inactive lifestyle limits attainment of optimal cognitive and brain health. These thoughts are also in accord with daoist findings on attainment of health and longevity.

Glenn A. Gaesser, Stephanie E. Hall, Siddhartha S. Angadi, David C. Poole, and Susan B. Racette in their 2025 article in Journal of Applied Physiology said that physical inactivity and excessive calorie intake occupy dominant roles both in health related problems, and by redressing them, in the relevant solution. They reviewed several sources and focused on evidence that appropriate exercise engagement and calorie restriction (CR) can improve physical and mental health with a view to extending the health span. They concluded that "Humanity, writ large, has grasped these underlying concepts for Millennia but has been largely intransigent to them", which basically means that humanity at large is guilty of ignoring the facts about their health throughout history and all over the planet in different cultures.

I like to point out that by the year 2030 elderly adults over 65 years of age is estimated to comprise 20% of the population, and by 2050 the number of people 60 years old and over worldwide to be 21.1% or 2 billion. Because of the increasing aging population in many countries throughout the world, much evidence shows that pharmacological treatment, in some instances, is indispensable during the aging process. However, a non-pharmacological approach can be just as effective if not more given it does not disrupt the normal bodily function of interest and be used in the prevention or management of the disease at hand. But people have to strt as young as possible to develop a de-institutionalized form of exercise and nourishment style that can be generational thought by the older to the younger to maintain and develop family health, and that has to protect the family, clan, or community against disease through periods of poverty, disaster, war etc. Health-Autonomy, or Health-independence, are here the magic words. General research usually starts and ends by organisations that maintain some form of control over the users of their programs, and that is why this book is here to help you gain autonomy, but also why the research is there to test how much of what people need to develop health autonomy. One thing that people need according to the research is that tghey need methods and understanding that can be accessed easily through a language rooted in that experience. Scientific lingo is usually about aspects of your body you cannot see or feel (even though some people with large imagination think they can).

Myocites for instance. Myocytes are muscle cells, the fundamental units of muscle tissue, responsible for contraction, at least in western muscle physiological theory. There are three main types in vertebrates: skeletal, smooth, and cardiac, each with specialized functions and structures, but all sharing the perceived common purpose of contraction and relaxation. They are essential for movement, organ function, and blood circulation.

Another example of scientific lingo is a rapportage or suggestion by the World Health Organization (WHO) considers both intensity for Physical Activity (PA) and also the frequency of weekly PA adjusted to age. Therefore, adults aged 18-64 yrs and for adults > 65 yrs are recommended a minimum seventy-five minutes of vigorous-intensity aerobic PA or at least 150 min of moderate- intensity aerobic activity per week, respectively. These recommendations are important to be considered since sedentary time and total Moderate-to-Vigorous (MVPA) activities are associated to health risk in adults. An equivalent combination of MVPA can be suggested, such as 2.5 hours of lawn-mowing t (21 min/day) or 75 min. vigorous biking (11 min/day) fulfills weekly PA energy expenditure recommended by WHO for human health as well. You can feel the intensity of what you do, and you can feel when you overdo and thus become tired, but you cannot measure your energy expenditure. You cannot even second guess it.

What we can do by using our senses is mindmapping our interior and thus scaling our perception to a degree. But the ability of our senses to self experience is not unlimited. Definately we can exercise our senses to notice details that might seem supernatural or paranormal to the untrained. We can achieve also physical abilities that seem supernatural to the untrained. These things take time. All useful growth is slow, incremental even.

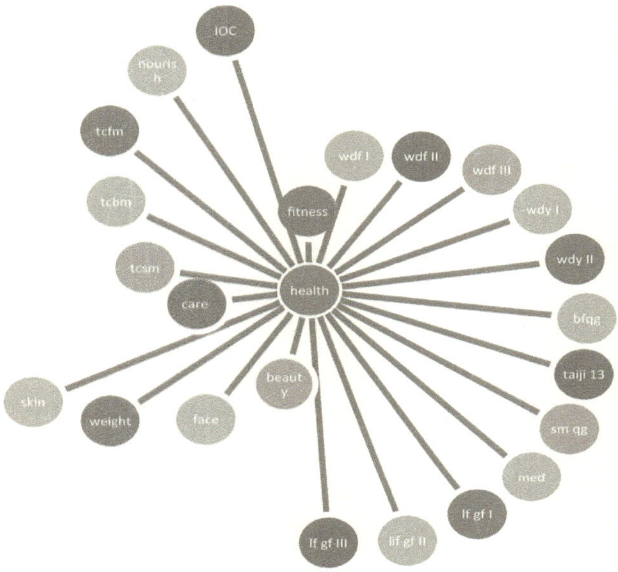

You always wanted to work on your health but never felt motivated or even felt demotivated due to the hard work and risks modern sports and medicine put you to without actually fulfilling promises? Then the Daoland Healthcare manual you are now facing is likely the answer to your problem. It explains you why you still get older and more worrysome, it shows you why puberty is hard for many, it shows you the level of nonsense found in many commercial self-help books, but most important, it shows you a way out of that running mill and into a rich life of self- generated brightness based on simple practical and cultural realism, looking at our neighbors and ourselves, nature and society. Starting to build your own personal global healthcare support program was never as easy as from today.

PART 7

My Seldon solution

1: The research program

From here we go focus on the content of the research. The text here in part 4 is brief, becasue of all the things we already explained. In the 2nd chapter I explain which subjects you get as a participant. In the further chapters I show you the principles above in the form of practical exercises you can do as a particpant on the research, or just to ad to your daily program.

One more time, I do hope that the book motivates you to belong to the first to get the full 3 skill program from which each individual skill normally on the commercial market will cost you a few hundred Euro's or USD to learn, if someone even offers it. All these skills are based on going through a timely learning curve. That curve should be 100 days minimum but can be extended to 6 months. To achieve this, participation will ask from you a dedication of 1-3 hours of self study per day, plus some additional focus group class moments and interviews. Before and after the research we ask from you to have a blood test and send in the results for later data processing. This will happen anonymously. But for biomedical research procf I need to show that there was a measurable effect. The outcomes of interviews and focusgroups etc is not considered valid enough for some purposes, so this is the way to counter it. It takes from you this as an investment as a stakeholder, plus a monthly membership, which can be offered with a discount if paid for as a year amount. That is the time I ask from you. You get each of these programs in drip format, that means that you get new parts every day or nearly every day as part of your earning program.

In this subscription form:

https://forms.gle/d4NWyARJ9C6Qodbf7

please fill in the link in your browser to access the form. I understand I ask a lot of you, but the participation will be worth the effort I am sure.

you are also asked how much time you can invest for 5 days per week minimum. You will likely get added to a group based on your available time. For the rest what classes you get appointed to is randomized, so neither you nor I can know this on forehand. It doesn't matter for the program if you like the program or not, the outcomes are hopefully representing a general expectation for a larger audience in their reception and effects, The test is divided in 8 groups for a 1000 participants:

1. *meditation*
2. *gongfu fitness*
3. *food medicines*
4. *meditation and gongfu fitness*
5. *meditation and food medicines*
6. *gongfu fitness and food medicines*
7. *meditation, gongfu fitness, and food medicines*
8. *random weekly classes with qigong, breathwork, taijiquan and yoga*

After the test cycle is over you can maintain your membership and have access to the programs not in your group. People after you will all get the same program but will only be tested randomly to measure longterm effects. We talk of years.

Most important of the exercise is to test you on how you implement it in your liofe and how your retention of the skills is. After the research is finished we hope to charter you as a Daoland Volunteer. Daoland Volunteers are what we call "Health builders", not just for themselves, but also for others/. After the big crunch has happened (if it does) people like you will become tribal organizers and healthcare providers, so the more you have learned within one systematic way of thinking the better. So you see, the research might lead to a wholy new career and life destiny. You remember the ide of being a good child and helping elder men and ladies cross the street?

Something like this. Societies always are in need of people who can help others to become healthy too. You should as a therapist or teacher always be a good example.

So let us discuss what the 3 programs are about in chapter 2.

2: Focus on 3 skills

As you have just read, in the research we focus on the three primary skills we think are most useful as survival skills to create health independence. These skills are going to be immedeately helpful in your daily life in that they ought to bring your healthcare costs down/ People who are vital, agile and have healthy feeding habits tend to be less likely to become sick or develop unhealthy signs of aging. Some reservations here, because before these exercises you might have a history with your health, so in that case the exercises have to become restorative. Maybe you have always eaten filling your desires, or large portions. Maybe your mind is always racing. In all these cases the exercises can be life changing. Life changing practices can alter your perspective on life.

The exercises are gfoing to be guided by me and my research assistants to help you getting the best outcomes.

meditation

- Meditation is commonly seen as a good practice to become mindful or to resolve stress related discomfort. But meditation is more complex than that. Just the idea that meditation is against stress or helps you to be mindful is a bit ridiculus. Yes on the long term it will those things, But meditation is also topsports. Just the sitting already can be quite a feat. In meditation you have to best sit on the floor in a vertical position in multiples of 25-30 minutes. This beginner stage is callt "the art of sitting" or "sitting skill", or "sit-battle". During this position we learn to hold our attention in a particular span of polarisation, which will be explained in the program. Every session comes with yogic preparation to help you reduce sitting stress. It also comes with a small focus ritual that you can do or do not do. That is up to you. In each session you get extra information to help you forward. What you do is cultivate yang. Yang is the warming and motivating factor of your body. It helps to moisten your body and battle aging. This yang will follow particular patterns in your body, which will be explained in the course. Since the course is focussed on 100 days of learning and then how you continue to incorporate it in your daily life and what benefits you experience, it is a rather complete program that has to teach you not only to cultivate yang, but also how to control yang. Like with everything in life, too much of a good thing is a bad thing.

food medicine

- Chinese medicine start with the idea that food is a teacher, that has to show you ways of existence that we can benefit from. The Food then is seen as an example of how things can be done, and by eating these things our body learns. You know the saying ÿou are what you eat"? The Chinesen also use a saying li<e that. Food changes you in sometimes unexpected ways. So doing these exercises have to make you aware of how that happens. It also provides you with several relevant details about food production, gives you some recipy ideas etc. The practices are simple and repetetive, not to give you as many experiences as possible, but to help you refine your taste so it becomes a useful tool in food selection, preparation and digestion. In many ways it is a form of meditation too. It teaches you to eat in relationship to your personal needs. When shared in a family all members can learn to make their own food selection. Little kids just eat with their parents to generate the right taste habits, but then eventually become more independent. A fun fat is that I learned this method from a Daoist herbalist who used to take me into the mountains, as part of a larger mediine learning system, likely going back to neolithic times, but certainly to Sun Simiao, in which School I have been initiated as a disciple (this means that I was accepted in a father-son relationship with my teacher). In China, being part of Sun Pai gives you a special status.

physical capacity

— As a Daoist we learn a lot about exercise. Mobility is the proof that you are a alive, and the more mobile you are , the more you are alive. And ofcxourse, when we are young moving is easy, although moving properly isn't as easy as it seems, so we tend to focus on the wrong kind of movements and with the wrong goals to move for in mind. In these Gongfu programs you learn to increase your agility and mobility. Once you can manage pretty fast agile movements and your range has become larger and larger you literally become younger. Taijiquan or Wushu isn't going to do it for you, neither is the gym. Becasue it isn't just about moving fast or strongluy or competetively, but it is in the work that we do while moving. We like to work less but work more. I think this is a nice paradoxical way of explaining things. So in the course where you learn some 120 exercises you have to learn to limit certain functions of the body, such as sweating behaviour, breathing behaviour, emotional behaviours, etc. Again this is sort of a meditative form of exercise, a meditation on movement so to say. The purpose is to become easy in movement and unstoppable, even on a high age. These are things no bicycle , earobics or yoga class will teach you.

3: Becoming a professional Human

The secret of life is a simple solution to the problems we experience in life. As such we need a learning program to show us what it means to be human in regard to the rest of nature. Not as being differentiated from nature and stricktly shielded against it, but in how we fit in with nature. We do so by understanding ourselves as nature.

The thing is, that the daily nature we see every day is entropic. This means that 'everything that rises must converge'. The problems with life are twofold:

1. Life is resisting life through inner friction, conflict if you wish. This inner friction is casued by things that we

eat, the oxination of our body from breathing, and the synthetic stuff that we drink or medicate ourselves with. Conservatives, preservatives, quasi paralitics all kind of stuff that mummify us and make us hold out longer, meaning, wrinkle less, but because of wrong care, suffer more while aging too.

2. Life is asymmetrical. This asymmetry is embodies in our inner body through the asymmetrical placement of our organs, while aparently outward we are symmetrical. Our feelings too are asymetrical. In Daoism and Buddhism alike we speak of two base states of feeling: the state of affinity and the state of aversion. The state of affinity seems familiar, but might not be. The state of affinity is the recognition of life in things. A car doesn't have it, and neiter do our clothes and kitchen implements. But a tree, a scorpio and a waterbear have it. When tribal people talk of an animated natere spirit, when we talk of Qi, or Ki in Japanese, and Gi in Korean, we speak of this natural perfection which is both harmonious, unspectacular and nearly unnoticed. People sometimes think love is like that, but it isn't. Affinity is indiscriminate. Love is discriminate. We have to look at aversion to understand love.

Aversion is based on three base instincts: anger, desire, and fea. These three rule all of our emotional life. I am sure some of the people reading this will trend to immedeately reject this. But daoism calles our emotions afflictions. There are seven of them and they are combined with the six desires.

The term "seven emotions" comes from The Book of Rites, referring to happiness, anger, sadness, fear, love, hatred, and desire. The term "six desires" first appeared in Master Lü's Spring and Autumn Annals, referring to human desire for life, desire against death, and the desires of human organs such as ears, eyes, mouth and nose for sound, color, taste and aroma. Later, the term "seven emotions and six desires" came to be used to describe people's emotions and desires in general. Such emotions and desires, being naturally born with people, should be released or satisfied as appropriate. But they should not become excessive.

Both these text are about 2500 years old, and in general they meant that these feelings create asymmetrical forces in our body, which we can determine to be feelings of potential or actual friction, also to be named 'energy outbursts'.

The sensations we feel in the body when doing exercises like meditation, visualisation, qigong or taijiquan are signs of friction and asymmetry. The task of dealing with them to achieve health and longevity is a lifelong task. In fact, what I like to say to any of my friends and students is that we as people have only one job, namely "being and staying alive". You may think that you need a job to stay alive, but in reorganizing our priorities we can work together to get the nescessary things to be done. As a result we can work on our self-cultivation and maximize our help as our major job. No tools required.

There are several apects to that. We will briefly discuss three:

4: Learning time and epigenetic conditioning

When cultivating health we need time to practice. When we learn proper practice when young, we can gradually gather all the skills and the normalcy as a society to embrace self-cultivationas a core medical practice. When aging it makes maintenance and permanent life The research I do wants to investigate it as a general possibility, but primarily it wants to understand how eager we are to control our health by ourselves, and how far that can bring us.

In modern Biology we see that we humans and other complex multicellular organisms, we all have systems of organs that work together, carrying out processes that keep us alive. The body also has levels of organization that build on each other. Chemicals make molecules, morecules build organelles, organelles make cells, cells make up tissues, tissues make up organs, and organs make up organ systems. Organ systems make the species. The individual expression of a part of the species. The function of an organ system depends on the integrated activity of its organs. For instance, digestive system organs cooperate to process food. The survival of the organism depends on the integrated activity of all the organ systems, coordinated by the blood, fascia, lympf, endocrine and nervous systems. As a general idea it is suggested that most of these processes are sort of organically automated. The digestion, the breathing, the blinking of our eyes, many functions seem to be out of our control in that way of thinking. Similar like it determined that our mind has huge parts out of our control. Daoist self-cultivation does not agree with that. It agrees that we are born with particular base settings. And we can live our whole life with that, grow old and die. But that is a narrow slith of life between the inanimate and the animate to be satisfy with. Self-cultivation wants to widen that narrow band by finetuning the mental and physical systems.

Through reducing the friction, taking body functions under conscious action, hacking it, so to say, we can overcome its tendency to gradually collapse.

To do so we need to figure each individually out how much time we need to get there. There are no standard values for that. But we can estimate that in the learning time per skill one hour per day is enough to begin with. The rest is dependent on your personal circumstances. Too much exercise will increase friction, and too little leaves it intact.

Modern science has first disvered the genes. The genes contain a sheer endless set of information instructing to become what we are. But the genetic is dependent on circumstances to express the ideal settings. Wrong circumstances generate disease, cancer, decay of the endpieces of our gene strings etc. Right circumstances do the opposite. That means that environment and behavior are great tools for healing and for aging. We call this epigenetic conditioning. This has been extensively investigated in Chinese research on qigong and exercise.

Epigenetic conditioning through exercise creates a "memory" in the genome by altering gene expression without changing the DNA sequence, which influences long-term behavioral and physiological adaptation. Exercise triggers epigenetic modifications like DNA methylation and histone changes, which are influenced by factors like mitochondria function and redox pathways, to regulate gene activity in areas such as muscle repair, metabolism, and brain function. These modifications help build a protective epigenetic memory that can reduce the risk of chronic diseases and improve overall health. That allows for an indeterminate destiny in life and the opportunity to age well.

In a 2012 article Hua Ren et al.[li] Showed that an increasing number of studies are pointing to physiological and psychosocial benefits of taijiquaqn and qigong in terms of improving quality of life and physical and physiological function including musculoskeletal strength, flexibility, cardiovascular fitness, and immune response. Other studies have shown that these offer therapeutic benefits for patients with chronic and debilitating conditions such as fibromyalgia, Parkinson's disease, rheumatoid arthritis, and osteoarthritis. However, the biological mechanisms by which taijiquan exerts its effects remain unknown, and there are no known biomarkers that can be used to determine the efficacy of taiji or changes that may accompany taiji practice at the molecular or cellular level. I can cite more sources. But I will at this point leave that for later. Epigenetic change still requires research and our research has to motivate that too, through our blood testing and through our questionaires etc.

5: Family management

A family is a growing entity over time. From generation people do not just exist accidentally, but they are the core of their species. They collect skills and qualities and they need to be passed from generation to generation. A child is becoming a human, a parent is a nurse, a doctor, and a teacher. This program is meant to be combined with another program that will come online at a later date. It is a module explaining how to raise health in kids, how to manage yourself in preparation of aging, how to stall aging bad, and how to enter the end stage of life. Combining it with the wildeness module not will give also the alchemical solution to not dying explained.

What is clear is that management of your family isn't that much different from managing a community, or society at large. It is organic and asymetrical, political and philosophycal. Personally I take a freedom based aproach to child education. But I am strict in my guidance and do push my children to improve themselves, to help them regulate their feelings, and to share skills for health they will need later if they want to use them. I also share the skills to teach and to heal with them when it is their time. They might reject it, and that is their choice to make. You cannot force children, as you cannot force the elderly to discipline themselves when already old, their worldview is frozen in time. But young people are more flexible. So when we learn these skills and share them with our kids, in a few generations there will be more and more lifelong involved people in natural community healthcare through proper life methodology. The proper family management set up buy practitioners will eventually lead to new forms of leadership and

6: Community building.

Community building is a task set up as a moral obligation for those able to do so. It is up to you how to do that. Eventually we can have a lengthy discussion on that together through an online forum.

7: The secrets of Composure

Our nature is determined by our outer form. Our body shape reveals our bodily ability and adaptability. This is what I earlyer explained as being shaped by the Jing, the cohering force inside our body. This force is shaped by our actions and our intent, guided by our awareness, that in turn requires an idea and a working theory on what to do to get to the goal of maximizing our body shape as to achieve maximized body function. The main goal is to generate internal volume by moving the parts more apart from each other, not so much by making them stronger or more swollen, as we do in regular sports. You understand where the word self-cultivation comes from. In Chinese medicine it is in essence suggested that we can regulate our social connections through our body posture, We all know that people with intense emotions deviate in posture from healthy people. With healthy people I do not mean the bulgy muscular people with swollen chest and seemingly ready to attack you. That is what we call warrior style. It is a sign of imbalenced hormones, and ill distributed blood. A good posture has relaxed hanging shoulders, the chest is neither flat not round or hollow. The belly lays in the bowl of the hips and is relaxed. The legs are straght, the arms as well. There is no clear tone in the muscles. Due to the relaxedness the body is filled but not overflowing. Depending on your body type there are variations. This book is not involved with that. A following book will adress that.

In Chinese Daoist medicine two great thinkers come forward. One is Huangdi, whom was both a warrior king and a students of healthpractices (Yangsheng). Many papers are produced over time attributed to him or based on the core writings from some 2500 years ago. Even more famous is Laozi who wrote a relatively small text of only 5000 characters but has been more widely read than the Christian bible or Koran. Hard to imagine right? The two are often summarized in the name combination "Huang-Lao school of thought", while in fact it should be the "Huang-Lao school of Medicine". Both in their own way were involved with health: health of the body, and health of the person in society. They both had a very different approach. Huangdi in essence was a numerologist. That means he did seek our numerical order in things, much like modern science does. He emphasized that regularity in lifestyle, adaptation to the rithms of nature, the patterns of the up and down flow of qi and blood in the channels are the essence of health. Laozi on the other hand emphasized that the placement of the person in the larger universal context made health and harmony was essential. Laozi also emphasized that being specialized in a particular action will make you weak. So a person practicing high level sports of a kind will be weaker than an evaraging generalist. A mathematician will risk her or his life more than someone who just knows basic calculus. Focussing on scientific accuracy is more dangerous for health than experiencing oneself and developing a general idea of how things work and can be influenced.

The combination of these two approaches is what is called Dan Dao Medicine. The root of Chinese medicine, including integrated self-cultivation and life, as well as the availability of tools and people who can help in case of more complicated issues, doctors, if you will. But then, a good doctor is not a specalist, but a generalist, that understands the patterns of nature through experience and can use that numerical logic to help restore harmony. For a doctor to be a self- cultivator, a meditative inner alchemist if you like, was the essence of Chinese/Daoist medical science before modern times. It was also seen as the best solution if that methodology was shared among the people, along with an awareness that each in the end is responsible for one's own health as part of the maturation process. The Wudang Daoist Zhang Sanfeng wrote about this to the Song Emperor, to start a process of public education of the civilian population. Unfortunately it never happened. But Zhang is still widely revered in China.

Sun Simiao (581–682) was a Chinese physician and writer of the Sui and Tang dynasty, who was from Tongchuan, central Shaanxi. The emperor gave him the title "King of Medicine" (藥王; 药王, Yaowang) for his significant contributions to Chinese medicine and tremendous care to his patients. He did write many articles and some of them got lost. He retreated into the mountains to study and practice clinical medicine. For therapists he suggested the study of Yijing, numerology, Daoism, Confucianism, Buddhism etc. He followed the wisdom of Huang-Lao. Huangdi had learned that the physician should treat every client as if it was a family member, and not because of its economic value. When you become Sun pai Dandao medicine person we follow that idea too. Sun explained it in his book "the great physician's sincerity" (not yet translated) as: "A Great Physician should not pay attention to status, wealth or age; neither should he question whether the particular person is attractive or unattractive, whether he is an enemy or friend, whether he is a Chinese or a foreigner, or finally, whether he is uneducated or educated. He should meet everyone on equal grounds. He should always act as if he were thinking of his close relatives", and: "When a great physician treats illness, he should first calm his mind and focus his will, be free from desires and wants, first develop a great compassionate heart, and vow to universally relieve the suffering of all living beings". Like all emperical scientists he also ordered physicians to only dispense medicine tried out on themselves. They should exercise, know nature, meditate, do ritual etc.[ii] All minds of stuff that is summarized in the westere saying: "Know thyself", although I do not think the content of knowing thyself is the same.

The idea was that we should learn to build health through the exercises in the lower dantian, make relationship with the world in the middle dantian, and break out of one's conditioning in the upper dantian through identifying and knowing the world around us. Through exercising ourselves we learn to keep ourselves composed. 'Composure' is an idea that is reverberating the idea of not being moved out of harmony by the things happening inside and around us. Composure gives us reaction time. The time of not immedeately reacting allows you to know which are real and which are apparent events, So that we do not react on everythinbg. Even mice have composure. When they see you they first stop and observe to come to a measure of danger. This is not in conflict with the idea of 'taiji', practiced by Daoists. Taiji is a state of direct knowing by having practiced something endlessly for the eventual incidence something is going to happen. The research and this book allows for Taiji, to practice skills that will help us age well, but will be necessities when disaster strikes. When disaster strikes we need to not panick, but if we do not have a suitable toolbox, not panicking isn't an option. Being frozen in fear also isn't a correct reply. If we think of taiji like this it is in mean ing close to the idea of 'intuition'. Intuition also is based on what we already know. With intuition we also need to separate 'having experience' from accumulation of experience leading to understanding. Intuition is a shortcut based on the second observation.

Perhaps we can say that taiji and intuition are quite similar. I do not dare to say they are the same. But I do know that due to cultiral drift, some people came to associate intuition with knowing things without having to study for it. Babies do not have intuition for sucking on a nipple to ingest milk without having to study it, but we as people have learned this over millions of mammal generation. It is born into us. Composure is caused by learned action that has overtaken other impulses for our benefit. Panick is the opposite, but due to repetetive action we also can have frequent panicking becoming a habit. Exercise has to overcome negative habits and replace them by positive habits.

8: Inner calm and health

Due to the exercise program we build natural confidence. Natural confidence creates inner calm. Many exercises we do are there to help us develop inner calm. The Daoist idea of inner calm is that it generates inner clarity, and inner clarity generates space to get more effect and benefit from doing exercise, which does help to produce proper inner functioning, proper relationship with nature and other people, all summarized as 'general health'.

Inner calm especially reduces our mental stress. Mental, physical, and social stress create heat and pressure in our head, reducing the receptivity for sense impressions. In our head blood accumulates, but pressure reduces the ability to get waste products from our brain, creating foggy minds, dizzyness sometimes too, and a variety of levels of desorientation.

Exercises as learning how to stand on your heals and feeling how your weight sinks is a simple trick to lower your blood pressure and to let both heat and pressure sink by bringing blood flow back to its original dispersed state. There is a but though, becasue when you close your eyes doing that you might fall over, or faint. That is usually due to too much lowering of blood pressure in your head. By keeping your senses open you are continuously recalibrating balance and pressure. You can imagine how this helps to keep your health in harmony.

What most people do not realize is that the effectiveness of our senses calibrate our inner wellbeing. In 2013 there was a research published just on that. [liii] They explained the idea of sensory plasticity, that is the success in which senses can correct themselves. They also made clear that when an organ gets less efficient, it gets no urgency to be recallibrated and its relationship with the interior does then not controibute to our well being. General physical wellness in turn helps to restore the senses, when damage hasn't become permanent that is. Much can be corrected medically or through operative intervention, acupuncture and exercise. But especially with medication addiction to medication can give nasty longterm risks, and operations also never restore towards the original. Past a certain point also for herbs, needles or exercise are not going to help anymore.

Meditation ofcourse is a great tool to hone your senses, but also agility fitness fitness training can do so. Food medicine helps you develop taste and smell, so within the research program all the senses are bing adressed to keep you up to the best state and keep the callibration going. All depends on deverlopin g inner calm. But what we note here is that it isn't the meditation in itself that generates inner calm, it is the subject that we meditate on that does so. Therefore one meditation isn't the same as another.

What we do know that calmth isn't only affecting your own behaviour and health. It also affects your role in your environment. People feel naturally unease araounbd, and attracted towards calm people. Unease becasue you seem so tense around that person, and attracted becasue you develop a natural trust in a calm person. Calmth is therefore not only a tool for health, but also a tool to develop leadership quality. In households where everyone is load and nerveous the risk for agressive conflict is much larger than in a housella where people are calm.

Emi Linds, a growth strategist who helps organizations move the only thing that ever moves markets, namely human behaviour, suggests in a 2025 article that just like I do myself explain already for many years that stress narrows the brain's executive capacity. Under threat, cortisol floods working memory, constraining judgment and language precision. Psychologists call this the threat-efficacy loop: when perceived pressure exceeds perceived control, cognitive flexibility declines.[liv] It basically comes down that adrenaline rush that naturally brings us in a fight-or-flight mode can degrade the very capabilities organization depend on: strategic foresight, composure in negotiations, and sound risk assessment.

In performance studies, composure consistently protects decision accuracy. Research showed that U.S. military personnel who received pre-meditative mindfulness training -and practiced regularly (high-practice group)- maintained significantly higher working memory capacity (WMC), an index of accuracy in high-pressure decision tasks, compared to both the control and low-practice groups.[lv] In corporate research, teams led by emotionally regulated leaders sustain higher creativity and working-memory capacity under deadline pressure, So you can imagine how under proper guidance you can benefit from such an approach too, especially in a high pressure situation as a natural disaster, living in a warzone, becomeing a refugee, or simply suddenly becoming extremely poor. You are ofcourse not helped by intense fear, regret, or anger. Not to have such feelings might be hard, but to regulate them so that you can function properly isn't that hard, with a bit of practice.

In an article at the online 'Center for Creative L eadership', they suggest that a good leader should have integrity, self-awareness, courage, respect, compassion, and resilience. They should be learning agile and flex their influence while communicating the vision, showing gratitude, and collaborating effectively. In this sense they are pretty much in line with the Daoland healthcare program and a lot of Daoist ideas.

9: Solution building

A big tasks for the Daoland Healthcare program has always been to generate progrtams for people to affect their own health in a positive way. In the book so far we have shown many aspects of that, and how you can affect your health positively with simple solutiions that can be passed down in a family or community from generration to generation as a parenting responsibility.

Parenting is something that comple,ments education. In the past all parenting was sharing survival skills with the next generation. That urge to survive is now mostly taken over by the convenience of modern life. And although living in this convenience seems eternal when we are in the now, the parental responsibility isn't over. We still need to safeguard ourselves against excessive risks, especially in this modern time with all the gradually developing riskfactors creeping up to you.

The research I have invited you to partake in makes you efficiently co-responsible for guiding yourself and your community through any kind of hard time. I am not talking about becoming a warrior or anything. I speak of doing the right thing at the right time, namely non-violently restoring normalcy in life of you and your community, involve people with that and build that out to restart the civil seeds of society. A friend of mine, when hearing about the book I am writing, said half jokingly: *"Ah, your Seldon Plan!?"* referring the "The Foundation" book series from the scifi writer Isaac Asimov (1920-1992). But he could also have referred to the book of Lewis Dartnell's 'The Knowledge", dealing with the tools you need to restart civilization after a cataclysmic event. [lvi]

Below I will briefly outline how the content of the research will benefit you in a few situations. If you have questions about your situation, just join the program to be able to ask all your questions, and getting them asnwered. I think the simple [prctices in this book should be implemented as a no brainer. Creating positive control over your health benefits your life in amazing ways. Sure, natural processes often are very slow, but some issues might find resolve superfast. And if they do , do not foget to keep on practicing. You always need to have a buffer zone in your health, this is called resillience.

10. Solutions for city life

To know your environment means to know your options. So let us explore some opportunities before we do anything about our health. Because you need to know what likely and unlikely dangeres you face. First of all, how urgent is danger for you? Is there a risk for civil war, or war with another country, are you free to move about or are you living in a political system that curbs your freedom to move around? Define what are the boundaries of your safety and the safety of your community. Are you involved in a risky line of work, could you get wounded and lose your income, what kind of social securities are there now, and what is the economic well being of your environment?

Poor areas are more likely places to meet disaster due to poverty. Poverty breeds diseases and hunger, civil or actual war also creates inaccessibility to food and healthcare/medicines.

Based on your situation you should prepare for eventualities. In my country for instance civil war isn't likely at the moment. I know people feel politically fired up, but climate disaster is likely to happen. But in the case that central authority falls apart, it is good to have some supplies to eat from, and have some skills to benefit from, and these are skills that allow you to be as much self sufficient as you can be.

In my case natural disaster will be flooding. So you need to know which high buildings there are to see refuge. But usually there will be some warning signs, so timely leaving would be better. You need a place elsewhere. If youleave last moment you will see that all the roads will be overfull of other refugees, and you will not get far. You will need to continue on foot, which will make you slow and vulnerable. To have an alternate place on high ground that is not part of a civil strife or war would be great. Currently these places are already rare. The risk is all around.

But to know how to find food and keep your body healthy are core skills. Learning about herbs, massage, simple body manipulations will make you helpful, but having understanding of democratization and socialization of communities also is. You need to be able to build aliances with people based on compassion and trust, because in every crisis there will be looters and other kinds of bullies, which are led by the new kings and dictators after cataclysms. So understanding how to safeguard what is left of your neigbourhood is important. Having a network is important too. Staying locked into your house isn't good. You need an overview of the people in your community that can do particular tasks, such as building, repair, finding food, taking care of guarding, hygiene, the elderly, education of the young, etc. When any risks comes over the horizon you ought to reach out to your neighbourhood, or block anmd make arrangements already to work together. Have supplies in food and water if you can. But in many cataclysms these will be without value. You will need to understand what trees and shrubs are edible and which not. Your participation in the research allows you to take big steps in this direction. I already teach my kids about that from a young age. In the food medicine program you learn to validate how food substances stimulate your health. But you will need to build an understanding of some aggriculture too, to learn to safeguard food supplies over a long time. Just eating from shurbs as a subsistence lifestyle is romantic from a holliday perspective, but it isn't that much fun if the rest of your life will be like that. You can start by growing vegetables in your guarden and understand what kind of pests you might have there, like slugs, mice, etc. On the other hand, if you are meatarian, you like to know which snails and other grubs can feed you and which slugs will make you sick. You might want to grow an insectarium to replace meat, or grow mice, for which you need food supplies. Try beforehand. It isn't as easy as it seems. Worms and ants are good nourishment.

Native Americans used to eat ants. In survival courses you learn to eat worms. I learned from Australian Aboriginals that Woodlice are very healthy and nourishing, and abundant. They are easy to grow by creating wet wood surfaces they can live under. They create fertile soil too. Worms open up the soil.

From the brief material above, it is clear that you want to have a plan ready. You want to have a risk plan and a security plan, you want a neighbour plan and a longterm rebuild plan. Hopefully you will never need it. There is a lot you might want to know, and you can already build a knowledge and skill system in your family . You do not need a nuclear bunker. Surviving your bunker without having at least a 1000 people to build society isn't going to be helpful. Surviving cataclysms or war in a city isn't an individual survival, or just your family. It is a survival for the largest well cooperating socially coherent group that is able and willing to provide well being for all its members but then by communal sharing, not by authoritatian owners of the goods.

What is important to understand is that when you are tied to alocation you will need to be able to source food locally, and that requires organisation, understanding the climate, the seasons etc. It will be easy to exshaust your supplies, and to empty the land you live on. But thinking forward on how to renew is the secret of survival. For your body it is the same. Nature is timeless and well timed, but it is also fragile, just like we are. We can be strong, but only if we organize life adapting to the locality where we are.

11: Solutions for refugees

Once you are a refugee there will be stages of refugee-ness. First of all there is the fleeing, and then the travelling. You come across many hindrances. Country boarders , fearful people, local conflicts etc. It may take a while to find a safe place. If you reach a refugee camp, you will find that these usually are very limited in what they can offer you. So organize yourself as refugees and planning to build socially and materially in that place is important. It isn't about building personal or family wealth, but it is a bout building community.

Refugee camps like Nakivale in Uganda and Meheba in Zambia have become thriving communities through a focus on entrepreneurship, community integration, and sustainable livelihoods. These successes are often driven by initiatives that provide vocational training, facilitate partnerships between refugees and host communities, and support refugee-led businesses that meet community needs and create economic opportunities.

In 2022, a collaborative reforestation initiative in partnership with the UNHCR, Lutheran World Federation, and Dutch National Postcode Lottery, was creating a Green Refugee Camp in Far North Cameroon. Successfully restoring 100 hectares around Minawao Refugee Camp, home to 63,000 refugees escaping violence from Nigeria, the project provides employment, shade, health benefits, and sustenance for hundreds of refugee and local families.

Beyond tree planting, the project replaces wood with locally produced eco-friendly cooking alternatives and swaps plastic tents with sustainable, regionally sourced shelters. Over 32,000 thriving trees in just over a year have revitalized Minawao's ecological balance, turning it green once again.[lvii]

After a global cataclysmnic event that support will not be there, but it gives a clear image of what you want to set as your ideal goal. Depending on your circomstances you need to set clear goals to where you want to move to. Greening and creating food surplus, healthy living and so on are achieved together over time. Do not get stuck in the present hoplesness.

12: Solutions for war victims

War victims are possibly the most traumatized people around. Current trauma management for war victims includes a multi-faceted approach that combines immediate medical care for physical injuries with long-term mental health support for psychological trauma. Medical management focuses on tactical care like controlling bleeding, managing airways, and addressing injuries with a tiered system of care that moves from the battlefield to advanced surgical facilities. Psychological and social support involves therapies like CPT (cognitive processing therapy) and EMDR (eye movement desentisization and Reprocessing), building resilience, and coping strategies such as talking to others and self-care.

Of course there are many situations possible where these are all not available. I bought a small opoeration kit, where I teach my kids with how to clean and repair wounds. Plants like calendula, turmeric, and tea tree oil are traditionally used to disinfect and heal wounds due to their antimicrobial and anti-inflammatory properties. Other plants include dill, yarrow, aloe vera, and centella asiatica, which can aid in wound healing by reducing bacteria, promoting collagen synthesis, and reducing inflammation. It is important to understand what plants in your environment can be used when common medical supplies are not available. You might need it for yourself, or for people around you.

Emotional trauma can last for a long time. PTSD, Post-traumatic stress disorder is a mental health condition that's caused by an extremely stressful or terrifying event, either being part of it or witnessing it. Symptoms may include flashbacks, nightmares, severe anxiety and uncontrollable thoughts about the event.

Self-treatment for PTSD involves a combination of lifestyle adjustments and coping strategies. In common society it is advised to combine it with professional treatment. But we do here deal with the assumption that that isn't available. The thing is that you do not wish to let it control your life and be part of the rebuilding of communal life, emphasis on communal. I beleive that being part of a scioal group that is supportive and shares goals is great medicine. Making yourself helpful in supporting others helps to whitewash the terrible situations you witnessed. In Nepal I had to hide behind a temple pillar during a shootout between rebels and the military, and in Bosnia I had the misfortune to come there just a few days after peace was made and trauma and wounds were everywhere all too visible. Another time I was with friends at a coke party in a squat and my friend sneezed, blowing up the cocaine in the air. We were thrown out of the party but not before i first got a pistal in my face with an upset face blaming me for the action. There were other things that could have been traumatic. But I think that helping other people has over time solved the emotional pressure of the situations I was in. Besides helping others, you can support your recovery by maintaining routines, engaging in stress-reducing activities like exercise, meditation, or yoga, and connecting with trusted friends, family, or support groups. Staying grounded with techniques like slow breathing or sensory activating meditations, avoiding alcohol or drugs, and being patient with yourself as symptoms gradually improve.

PTSD was one of the considerations in developing the research. It can be a destabilizing force in life as we go through any traumatic change. Even just divorce or disease and aging can cause trauma of sorts. The research project helps to create the kind of order and inner peace you need for PTSD. The breathing, preparatory yoga, and meditation helps (as you know from above) to calm your nerveous system and to open up your sense organs. The gongfu fitness routines help you to build resillience and detach action from breath contraints. Stress winds itself through our movements in the form of creating erratic moves, agression, edgy moves, lack of coordination. The unwinding eases back in control. The food medicine helps to selct foods that work for you and make it easyer to stay away from harmful toxins.

FINAL

Conclusions

I think that was about it. I think I have said the most of it. More will come after the conclusion of the research, Please follow the link here to join the research as a stakeholder. Be motivated and in eventuality, become a force for good:

The link: https://forms.gle/d4NWyARJ9C6Qodbf7

Conclusion and a words of thinks

First of all I should thank the many people who support me in my work. Without the people believing the things I say or being willing to test them, this book would never been written.

Thank you for the history that brought us at this intersection of knowledge systems and the technology to disseminate ideas fast and broadly. For the first time we have the opportunity to all think about humanity and we can make choices for our futures based on the myths and reams of our many pasts. They all teach us that being human equals being good people.

Thank you for reading my book, I hope you will enjoy a long and happy life. Hopefully one day soon we will meet and discuss the effects you had from implementing Daoland principles and how it altered the way how you embrace your own culture and landscape. I am sure it will help you enjoy the inherent wisdom/knowledge based values of your culture more. I think we are all parts in a larger research plan for increasing our success as a species and as guardians for the other creatures on this planet. We need to protect them mostly against our forgetting being human and the many ways of being good people.

In this book we discussed the risk assesment of the modern time. I made a proposal to build a generational healthcare, effectively splitting the healthcare away from the commercial economics of a healthcare of inequality. I also emphaisized that community building has to be at the core of every society, as does social equality, democratic rights and proper distribution of the results of group think and group work.

The core of the book is to tip you off on what you need to know about yourself and your environment to safeguard yourself against poverty, disaster, war, conflict etc. Has it become a survivalist manual? I think it has become a more realist version of these things. Survivalism is an expression of individualism in survival. But I do think that isn't available for the larger population. We are not as individualistic as we like to think. But if you are well prepared and are able to foster knowledge, skills and goodness, I think you are suitable material to guide future communities towards a start back into prosperity. We are all adventurers of sorts, but the adventure is to find health, peace and community.

The final goal of this book was to invite you to become partner in my research and take part in my own activism. As a future community we can achieve a lot. We can even chance the present. I do not know if we can avoic climatic change and disaster, but I am sure we can handle living with it. Perhaps we can support change in society by preparing ourselves healthwise, become more independent for this, develop it within our communities and share it with next generationsn and neighbouring social groups and cultures. We now know the world is far too small for conflicts and mineral exhaustion. The risks for living out in space isn't very attractive, because it will include sensory deprivement and poverty as well. Ofcourse humanity will make its own choices, but making choices to make life here better are always the best, because not everybody can live in bunkers or spaceships.

For this book I go to end this adventure and enter the adventure of the research itself. I also look forward to write more books. I have a list of topics. Below you will a link to page that shows you how to sign up for other courses that I give.

Rene Goris, my Wudang Daoist name You Li Ou.

11-11 2025

i. https://www.patreon.com/Daoland_Healthcare
ii. https://www.youtube.com/@daolandhealthbuilding and https://www.youtube.com/@Daoland-Everywhere
iii. Daniel Keyes, Hussein Turfe, Joe M. Das. Prevention Strategies. In: StatPearls [Internet]. Treasure Island (FL): StatPearls Publishing; https://pubmed.ncbi.nlm.nih.gov/30725907/. 2025
iv. Xü Anlong (editor in chief) . "Yinyang You: Biohacking with ancient codes". World Affairs press, Beijing, 2022
v. Wu Guozhong. Big Medicine, the Body has its Own Medicine. 武国忠. 人体自有大药. Nanjing Literature and Art publishing house, Nanjing. 2008
vi. Jingcheng Dong. 'The Relationship between Traditional Chinese Medicine and Modern Medicine'. 2013
vii. Syed Amin Tabish. 'Complementary and Alternative Healthcare: Is it Evidence-based?'. 2008.
viii. Andrew Chesterman. 'Contrastive Functional Analysis'. 1984.
ix. Marc Edelman et al. Food Souvereignity". "the Peasant Journal". (2014).
x. 神农: 著, 刘希茹: 今译, 孙星衍: 考据, 李照国: 英译. 神农本草经英译 Shanghai Sanyuan Bookstore/ (Englih bilingual Agriculture God's Canon of Materia Medica. 2022.
xi. Michel Foucault. "Birth of the Clinic: An archeology of medical Perception". Vintage, New York. 1994
xii. https://www.nri.cam.ac.uk/
xiii. Hing Keung Ma. " The Development of Altruism with Special Reference to Human Relationships". 2017.
xiv. Raquel Sánchez Recio, Juan Pablo Alonso Pérez De Ágreda, María José Rabanaque, and Isabel Aguilar Palacio. "Understanding the Effect of Economic Recession on Healthcare Services: A Systematic Review". the Iranian Journal of Public Health. 2022.
xv. https://youtu.be/zQThHCB_aec?si=dhoNohkmFJWSZEdf@DrMyrianFransois. "We have 900 days left" 22-11- 2025.
xvi. https://www.ioufoundation.org/
xvii. https://universidadazteca.net/
xviii. Here is referenced: Rene Goris: A tool for Learning, Onderzoek naar Qigong en Qigong gebaseerde Geneeskunden 2006 Master thesis IOC foundation, current at Aztec University, Mexico, summary in English
xix. Michael J. Winkelman: An Ethnological Model for Assessing Social Evolution of Siberian Shamans . 2024. Journal: Social Evolution & History. Volume 23, Number 1
xx. C M Hughes, J C McElnay, G F Fleming: Benefits and risks of self medication (2001) Drug safety, NIH, Springer Link
xxi. Koenig, Harold G.: Religion and Medicine I: Historical Background and Reasons for Separation. 2000/2001, International Journal of Psychiatry in Medicine; London
xxii. LEE, Youngsub; KIM, Hyoungsup: The Turning Point of China's Rural Public Health during the Cultural Revolution Period: Barefoot Doctors: A Narrative Review Article (2018) Iranian Journal of Public Health; Tehran
xxiii. Shenglang Tang: The Westernization of Traditional Chinese Medicine Hospitals in China: What needs to be done? 2012, https://globalhealth.duke.edu/news/westernization-traditional-chinese-medicine-hospitals-china-

what-needs- be-done, and Jingcheng Dong: The Relationship between Traditional Chinese Medicine and Modern Medicine. 2013, Hindawi Publishing Corporation: Evidence-Based Complementary and Alternative Medicine, Volume 2013,

xxiv. Jia-Chen Fu: Health and Medicine in Modern China. 2022, Oxford Research Encyclopedia; Asian History

xxv. Review: The Evolution of Health Care Systems in England, France and Germany in the Light of 1848 European Revolutions, Acta Sociologica Vol. 26, No. 1 (1983), pp. 83-88 (6 pages) Published By: Sage Publications, Ltd.

xxvi. Report of a WHO global survey: National policy on traditional medicine and regulation of herbal medicines. 2005, Geneva

xxvii. https://scholar.harvard.edu/files/mankiw/files/economics_of_healthcare.pdf

xxviii. Denholm, Bonnie. The Official Voice of Perioperative Nursing; 2012, AORN Journal: Denver Vol. 96, Iss. 2.

xxix. Joseph Needham, Lu Gwei djen: Biology and biological technology: Medicine, 2000, Science and Civilization in China volume 6 part 4, edited by Nathan Sivin, Cambridge University Press

xxx. Tummers, L.G. Explaining the willingness of public professionals to implement new policies: A policy alienation framework. (2011) International Review of Administrative Sciences,

xxxi. Gifford H. Millera, Richard B. Alley, Julie Brigham-Grette, Joan J. Fitzpatrick, Leonid Polyak, Mark C. Serreze, James W.C. White: Arctic amplification: can the past constrain the future? 2010, Elsevier, Science Direct, Quarternary science review,

xxxii. Matthias Garschagen, Michael Hagenlocher, Deepal Doshi, Jonathan Reith: Global patterns of disaster and climate risk—an analysis of the consistency of leading index-based assessments and their results. 2021, Springer, online presentation

xxxiii. https://nhess.copernicus.org/articles/25/287/2025/

xxxiv. Kevin D. Lafferty: The ecology of climate change and infectious diseases. 2009, Ecological Society of America, volume 90, issue 4

xxxv. https://thinkgrowth.org/the-doom-boom-inside-the-survival-industry-s-explosive-growth-2fece1f6cd6c, 2016.

xxxvi. Marjukka Parkkinen: Engagements with uncertain futures – Analysing survivalist preparedness. 2021, Finland Futures Research Centre, University of Turku, Turku School of Economics.

xxxvii. https://health.ec.europa.eu/health-security-and-infectious-diseases/overview_en

xxxviii. https://health.ec.europa.eu/health-emergency-preparedness-and-response-hera_en

xxxix. Benita E. Cohen, PhD,1 Annette Schultz, PhD,1 Elizabeth McGibbon, PhD,2 Madine VanderPlaat, PhD,3 Raewyn Bassett, PhD,4 Kathy GermAnn, PhD,5 Hope Beanlands, MN, MPA,6 Lesley Anne Fuga: A Conceptual Framework of Organizational Capacity for Public Health Equity Action (OC-PHEA). 2013, Can/Public Health 2013;104(3):e262-e266.

xl. Education as a Social Determinant of Health. 2021, https://publichealth.tulane.edu/blog/social-determinant-of- health-education-is-crucial/ 2021, Celia Scott Weatherhead School of Public health and Tropical Medicine xli. https://www.york.ac.uk/news-and-events/news/2018/research/neanderthal-healthcare-practices-key-to-survival/ 2018, University of York, UK

xlii. Ram Rajasekar, Sripathi Kandula: Zoopharmacognosy. 2008, Research Gate, Resonance magazine 13

xliii. Michel Foucault: Birth of the Clinic; an archeology of medical perception. 1963, translated in english by A.M. Sheridan, Routhledge publishers, London and New York

xliv. Thomas Kuhn: the structure of scientific revolutions. 1962, 1970, University of Chicago,

xlv. https://www.bprhub.com/blogs/iso-certification-baldrige-award-comparison#:~:text=ISO%209001%20focuses%20specifically%20on,including%20leadership%20and%20strategic%20 planning

xlvi. https://health.ec.europa.eu/eu-health-policy/overview_en

xlvii. https://www.thwink.org/sustain/glossary/KuhnCycle.htm, https://www.lri.fr/~mbl/Stanford/CS477/papers/Kuhn-SSR-2ndEd.pdf

xlviii. Nathan Sivin: Chinese Alchemy, preliminary studies. 1968, Harvard Monographs in the History of science, Also elaborated in Joseph Needham, Nathan Sivin: Science and Civilisation in China volume 6: Biology and Biological Technology part IV: Medicine. Cambridge University press

xlix. https://www.medicalnewstoday.com/articles/319532

l. https://yaledistilled.sites.yale.edu/browse-issues/2020-issue/biology-poverty-trap-how-genetic-modifications- perpetuate-socioeconomic

li. Hua Ren, Veronica Collins, Sandy J Clarke, Jin-Song Han, Paul Lam, Fiona Clay, Lara M Williamson, K H Andy Choo. 'Epigenetic Changes in Response to Tai Chi Practice: A Pilot Investigation of DNA Methylation Marks'. Evidence Based Complement Alternative Med. 2012 https://pmc.ncbi.nlm.nih.gov/articles/PMC3375016/

lii. Li Lixian, Tang Daocheng. Sun Simiao, the Medicine King: Daoist Yangsheng. Da Zhen publishing house co.ltd, Taipei. 2011-2018

liii. Adam Zaidel, Wei Ji Ma, Dora E Angelaki. 'Supervised calibration relies on the multisensory perception'. https://pmc.ncbi.nlm.nih.gov/articles/PMC3872253/ 2013

liv. Emi Linds. 'The science of calm: why composure is a leadership skill'. https://emilinds.ca/the-human-margin/the- science-of-calm-why-composure-is-a-leadership-skill/ 2025

lv. Jha, A. P., Stanley, E. A., Kiyonaga, A., Wong, L., & Gelfand, L. 'Examining the protective effects of mindfulness training on working memory capacity and affective experience'. Emotion Magazine nr 10 (2010).

lvi. Lewis Dartnell. 'The Knowledge: How to rebuild a civilization in the aftermath of a Cataclysm'. Penguin books, 2014

lvii. https://landlifecompany.com/projects/building-a-green-refugee-camp-with-unhcr

www.ingramcontent.com/pod-product-compliance
Lightning Source LLC
Chambersburg PA
CBHW031320230926
51848CB00001B/26